D0807419

I Want To Live

Gastric Bypass Reversal

Blessed Be
Dani Hart

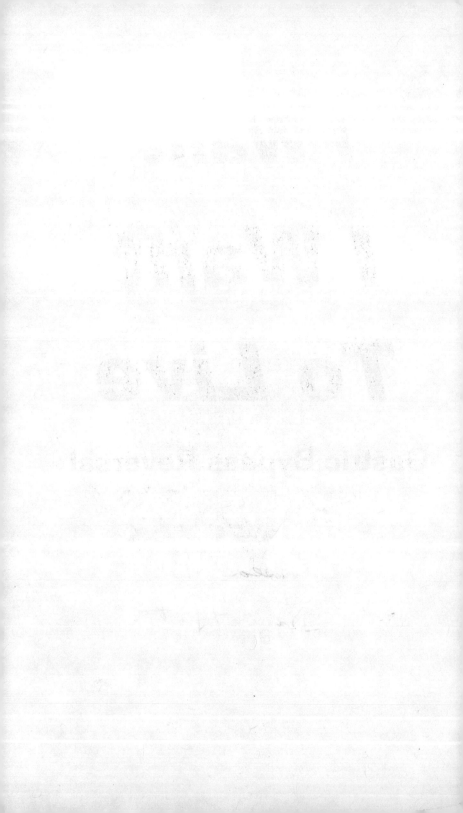

I Want To Live

Gastric Bypass Reversal

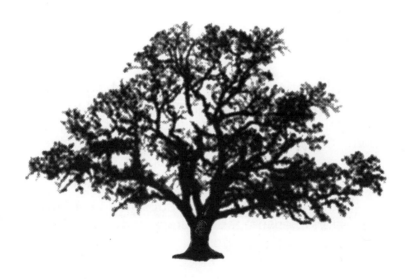

by Dani Hart

Published by Mountain Stars

Library of Congress Control Number: 2002115874

ISBN 0-9726554-0-9

Copyright © 2003 by Mountain Stars

First edition

Published by:

Mountain Stars
P.O. Box 270607
Fort Collins, Colorado 80527-0607

Printed in the United States of America using recycled acid-free paper.

All rights reserved. No part of this book may be reproduced by any means or in any form whatsoever, electronic or mechanical, including photocopying, recording, or by information storage and retrieval system – except by a reviewer or newspaper – without permission in writing from the publisher.

Although the author and publisher have made every effort to ensure the accuracy and completeness of information contained in this book, we assume no responsibility for errors, inaccuracies, omissions, or any inconsistency herein. Any slights of people, places, or organizations are unintentional.

All mail addressed to the author is forwarded, but the publisher cannot, unless specifically instructed by the author, give out an address or phone number.

Dedication

To those people who have had weight loss surgery and have passed on from complications associated with the procedure.

To those patients who are presently experiencing physical and emotional problems resulting from their weight loss surgery.

To those people who will decide to have the surgery in the future. My wish is that they will be well informed before making a life altering decision to have the surgery.

Acknowledgements

My children and husband have been through a lot with me during this journey with the weight loss surgery and the reversal. I will always be grateful for their support and willingness to help me. My family sacrificed a lot for me and has no regrets. They only want me to be happy and healthy.

To my sisters, brothers, and friends that stood by me throughout the hardest time in my life. They never abandoned me and provided love and compassion. I will forever be thankful they are in my life.

I thank my therapist who helped me prepare emotionally for the reversal surgery.

I am grateful for my family physician and Dr. Compassion who never gave up on me when I was so sick.

Thank you to Sue Widemark for all her assistance in providing information and support. Sue works tirelessly to help others, sharing her knowledge and empathy to anyone in search of help. You can see more about her web site and support group on the reference page.

My love will always go to the Goddess Mother Earth and the Great Spirit who showed me my strength lies within and that I had the courage to fight for my life.

Book Cover

The cover of my book represents the Tree Of Life

The Tree goes through cycles of growth

The roots of the Tree reaches deep within Mother
Earth for nourishment

The Tree provides a home for the birds and other
animal beings

The Tree represents strength but will bend in the
wind

The Tree is beautiful just the way it is

The Tree represents all of us

Dani Hart

Table of Contents

1

Introduction

From the day I first heard about the gastric bypass procedure to the present I have kept a journal detailing my personal journey. I am a very private person and it took a great deal of soul searching to decide whether to write it for others to read or to try to forget about all that has happened. I know others who have gone through a difficult experience with their Weight Loss Surgery (WLS) and wish to remain private, and I respect that.

I began writing about my experience with the gastric bypass surgery and the reversal procedure for my own healing process, which includes the mind, body and spirit. There are others that have gone through what I have and could relate to my journey.

My intent is not to persuade others to "have or not to have" a WLS, but rather to provide important information before they make a life altering decision.

At the time I began researching the gastric bypass surgery I believed the information provided by my doctor's office, people on a calling list provided by my doctor, and some of the online support groups, was sufficient enough to make a decision. After having the surgery and going through many problems I soon learned that I wasn't informed enough, or I would have never decided to have the gastric bypass surgery. The doctor's office I went to gave me a list of a few problems that could occur but left out so much information. The doctor minimized any problems that might occur by saying that I didn't need to worry about these, and that they seldom occur. I felt betrayed after learning there is so much more that could go wrong and that I had been misinformed about this from those I had spoken with before surgery. Anyone considering the gastric bypass surgery or any other weight loss surgery has a right to be informed of all the risks associated with these procedures. WLS patients deserve access to data on all the choices of weight loss surgeries. This information is not always available and some doctors may be reluctant to disclose statistics about complications and death rates.

Some patients have a good experience while others do not with the gastric bypass surgery. There is no way to tell ahead of time which category you will fit in. For myself, I feel the gastric bypass surgery gave me the ability to starve myself, and almost to death. I also ended up with multiple physical and emotional problems after the surgery that I never experienced before.

I am not a doctor, nor do I profess to know all about the medical pros and cons to the gastric bypass surgery or any WLS. *If you have any medical questions you should always consult your doctor.* I only know from my own experience and what I have learned from many others. I quickly learned that I was not alone with deteriorating health problems due to the RNY gastric bypass surgery.

I wanted the RNY gastric bypass surgery to work and did everything I was advised by the doctor who performed my surgery, but could not pretend my health was going well any longer. Several months after having the gastric bypass surgery my health had deteriorated to the point I became clinically depressed and contemplated taking my own life to end the suffering. Additionally, I experienced chronic vomiting and nausea, causing malnutrition which can lead to an early death. My family physician told me that I had 5 or less years to live if I did not have my surgery reversed. I felt I had a year or less to live at the rate my health was deteriorating.

At my lowest point I could not see a way out of the downward spiral that my life had taken. With the help of family, friends, and a strong will to never give up, I made a decision that would turn my life around for the positive.

The first step was to look within myself and make the choice to live or let life go. I chose life; *I wanted to live* and would fight to regain control. The second step was to seek help to see what options I had available and how I was going to go about making them happen. I sought help from my family physician; naturopath, psychologist, and a surgeon who would help me obtain a reversal (or takedown) of my gastric bypass, the RNY/Fobi with a silastic ring.

I reviewed all the options available and came to a very important decision to have my gastric bypass reversed. It was time to put balance back into my life, to enjoy doing activities with my family, and most important was to be physically and emotionally well. I do not believe there are mistakes, only opportunities to learn and to move forward. Having my gastric bypass reversed was a long and thought-out decision and by no means taken lightly. I did not want to go through another surgery, but under the circumstances with my chronic problems it was the best choice for me.

There are those who have had the surgery that would sacrifice anything in order to look better, and that was never my goal. I had the gastric bypass surgery to prevent future health problems, not to just fit into smaller clothes. The gastric bypass did not improve my health and quality of life, but rather caused all aspects of my life to deteriorate. Losing 130 pounds was not worth what I had to go through.

There are people who are satisfied with their gastric bypass surgery, and their stories are out for the public to read and watch on television programs. What I found missing is any downside to the procedure and felt it important that people considering this surgery have both sides of the surgery, the pros and cons. There are positive results regarding the gastric bypass surgery on the internet, doctor's offices, testimonials from people, and on-line support groups. My story will reveal what happens when the gastric bypass surgery does not work and what I went through to get my health back.

The names I use in my story are not the real names of the doctor's, friends, family, or others to protect their privacy. I will use names that I feel reflect the energy of the person. The doctor who performed my gastric bypass will be called Dr. No. I gave him this name because he had told me that the surgery could be easily reversed if I developed any health problems but later refused to help me. After having the Roux-en-Y (RNY) surgery and becoming very ill, Dr. No refused to even talk about reversing my gastric bypass. My story is more about the fact that this very invasive serious surgery of the gastric bypass can affect individuals differently. Some can have a great experience with it and others, like me, can find themselves, pretty soon in the game, slowly dying from it.

Integrity and honesty is very important to me so the truth will be told about my experience and from those who wished to share their stories.

2

Gastric Bypass

Surgery Decision

As a child I wasn't overweight, probably due to the fact I was a gymnast and worked on a farm. A high activity level was a way of life and still is. Obesity runs in my family and six out of seven sisters and brothers have problems with gaining weight very easily. Once we became older the weight seemed to stay on our bodies, no matter how active we were. Like other families, genetics plays a role in weight gain in my family. The ability to lose or maintain weight requires very little calorie intake for each of us. My father was a large person yet I very seldom saw him eat; we inherited his ability to utilize food efficiently.

My father took care of me and my siblings before he passed on at the age of 44 due to a heart attack. He had custody of us after my parents divorced, and after he passed on we went to live with relatives. I worked 16 hours a day at a restaurant and went to high school before putting myself through college. Working at a restaurant enabled me to have one meal a day. I went from riches to rags overnight, but there are no regrets with the path my life took. I became strong and self-sufficient.

When I entered into my twenties I started having problems keeping the extra pounds off, even though I wasn't eating very much. I would watch my roommate eat all she wanted and still stay thin as a rail. I wanted to be like her and eat normally, but that has never been the case. I thought I had been given a raw deal, getting inherited genes that put weight on my body by just smelling or looking at food. I know I chose this life for a reason and needed to find out why I needed extra weight and what I was going to do about it.

My weight started increasing after having children and even more so after having a complete hysterectomy. The hormone replacement therapy added over sixty pounds in one year so I went off of them and went to herbal remedies. I did not gain any more for quite some time, but I did not lose either. Being an obese person did not stop me from leading an active life and I climbed a mountain with an elevation around 14,000 feet. I was slow but made it, and was determined to continue to be as active as possible. Even though I tried to be active, I worried I would end up with physical complications when I got older like my father had.

Over the next few years my weight increased and it became frustrating to gain even though I still kept my calorie intake to around 1,500 calories a day. I kept a record of food intake and daily exercise to see what I was actually including in my diet. I tried many diets, as many of us have, and they did not work. I once lost 75 pounds by going down to 300 calories a day and working out two hours daily. Once I lost the weight, I had to stay at 500 calories to maintain my weight. An injury stopped my workouts and I gained back very rapidly. The years went by and my weight kept going up. Doctors told me to eat less and exercise more which I did, but the weight still did not come off. Many doctors feel that if you eat around 1,200 calories a day one should lose weight but that doesn't fit with everyone. I didn't want to go back down to 300 calories a day again. It was unhealthy and I was starving. A couple of doctors said I had one of the most efficient bodies when it came to utilizing food and that I would most likely outlive those in countries where there is very little to eat and still be overweight. That was not very encouraging but I never gave up at keeping active, nor did I slow down and become a couch potato.

I never binged in my life, even though I have thought about it, it just was not worth eating so many calories and not able to wear them off. Weight loss was hard enough without going up several pounds in a week from overeating. I also didn't want to become bulimic and ruin my body from vomiting. I have two siblings who became bulimic to lose weight and it has done damage to their bodies. They now have it under control and have found that eating smaller amounts of healthier foods along with exercising is the way to live healthier.

Weight gain was frustrating, but not the most important concern I had. A doctor told me weight gain can lead to physical problems down the road and if I didn't get it under control I would probably live less than five years the way I was. With a family history of obesity I wanted to look into other ways of getting the weight off to prevent complications in the future. I haven't found a doctor yet who didn't tell an obese person they had less than five years to live if they stayed overweight. There is no proof of this statement yet it is told to people who are overweight.

One day I was watching a television show about the gastric bypass surgery with a famous celebrity telling their story about weight loss and how happy they were. They never mentioned they had any major health problems after having the surgery so it was very encouraging to look into the procedure. The gastric bypass surgery seemed so simple and without problems. I read an article in the newspaper about a doctor in my area that performs these procedures and it all sounded wonderful. I thought that this might finally be a way for me to lose weight permanently, and be able to eat more than 300 calories a day to lose weight.

I began looking on the internet for more information regarding the gastric bypass surgery to see if others had been able to lose weight and keep it off. I soon found out there wasn't any information regarding the down side to the procedure, only a lot of information regarding the positive benefits. I thought the weight loss surgery must be the best thing in the world to lose weight and keep it off permanently. I had no information to think otherwise at that point in my search for the truth about the surgery.

With this information I decided to let my husband in on what I had been thinking of doing and why. I had not told him prior to my research because I wanted to have as much information about the gastric bypass surgery so we could sit down and go through it together. He knows how I have struggled with weight so he agreed with me to set up a consultation with the local doctor doing the Roux-en-Y surgery to get more information.

During my two month wait for the consultation appointment with Dr. No, I kept looking for anything about the gastric bypass surgery. I checked out an internet chat room for people who have already had the surgery. They all were so excited about it and had positive things to say. I noticed some brought up problems they were having, but were told it was either normal or that they must being doing something wrong. For example: eating sugar, drinking with meals, eating too fast, or not getting in enough protein and supplements. If someone was having problems then it had to be something they were doing wrong and it wasn't the surgery itself. At no time was it ever mentioned that there could be a problem with the weight loss surgery the person had. The comments in the chat room left me with the impression that if there were any complications it was the persons fault and not the surgery. I felt I would wait until I spoke with Dr. No before making a decision and counted on him to answer my questions and concerns.

Dr. No's office staff instructed me to attend one of their support groups meetings prior the consultation appointment. I went one evening to listen and hopefully learn more from people who had already had the surgery. Many of the people there told me Dr. No was one of the best in the country, has patients from around the world, and I should feel fortunate to have him do my surgery. Dr. No is also a member of the ASBS (American Society for Bariatric Surgery) and I had no reason to doubt his abilities as a doctor so felt confident going to the consultation in a few weeks.

The day came for my consultation visit and it included; filling out forms and questionnaires, taking my height and weight, watching a video about the procedure, and then about a ten minute consultation with Dr. No.

Dr. No said that I qualified for the procedure and would send his recommendation to my insurance company. He said his office is very good at getting insurance approval so it should not be a problem. Dr. No also told me the weight loss was permanent and I wouldn't have to worry again about gaining weight. This sounded wonderful to me; eating more than 300 calories a day to lose weight, and being able to keep it off permanently. Dr. No also told me I would be much healthier after the surgery and happier.

My surgery date had been scheduled, and within a few weeks of my consultation I received a letter letting me know the surgery had been approved by my insurance company. It actually surprised me that I was quickly approved since I did not have reflux disease, incontinence, diabetes, or sleep apnea, however, I did fit in the category of a BMI over 40, so I didn't question it any further. I trusted Dr. No to know what was best for me from a medical standpoint.

One of the most important statements Dr. No had said was, "if down the road you do not like having this surgery or have any medical problems it can be easily reversed", and this statement was reassuring. I knew that if something went wrong I could be put back the way I was before having the gastric bypass surgery. I did not anticipate anything going wrong and had a positive outlook. Dr. No told me that by watching his video about the surgery and reading the material he gave me I was well informed before going into the surgery.

Dr. No told me he would be doing the Roux-en-Y/Fobi (RNY) pouch with a silastic ring around the bottom of the pouch. At that time I was not aware of any other types of WLS, for example, the lap band. Dr. No had only told me about the RNY. There are many different options to choose from, but this is the procedure he does on his patients. (See Chapter 21 - Comparison of WLS Procedures).

Dr. No gave me a calling list of prior gastric bypass patients that I would be able to contact. I called several people on the list; a few did not want to talk about it at all and others talked freely. One woman in particular, I'll call Pat, went on and on about how wonderful the surgery was. She did not say one thing negative and strongly encouraged me to have the surgery. I spoke with Pat for several hours over the next few weeks leading up to my surgery. I asked many questions and kept getting the same response from her, "have the gastric bypass surgery". I spoke with several others on the calling list, and they were enthusiastic as well. So I felt I had first hand knowledge and the truth about what to expect.

I told my children, who were in their late teens, about the surgery I was about to undergo. They were unhappy about the decision and felt strongly that I should not go through with it. I told them of my concerns with my weight, how my father had died at a young age because of a heart attack, and that I was concerned I would have one as well because my doctor told me I might. I had always taught my children to follow their intuition and here I was not listening to them. I realize now that I was also not listening to my own intuition. I felt the surgery was going to improve my health, so I put it out of my mind about what my inner voice was saying regarding not going ahead with the surgery. At the time, I felt I was just being nervous about going into surgery and really believed what the people on the calling list told me was true and in the chat room. I had no reason not to believe them at that time.

3

Surgery Day and

Recovery

A week before having the Roux-en-Y surgery I had blood tests, an EKG, a pulmonary test, and a meeting with the nutritionist. I was suppose to have one hour with the nutritionist, but was delayed by other tests and ended up with only twenty minutes. I received hardly any information and was told to read over the information from Dr. No's office and that would be enough to prepare for what I could eat after the surgery. Dr. No and his nurse also reassured me they would be there to answer any questions and the nutritionist would be helpful as well.

My surgery day had arrived and I was prepared, or so I thought, for a new life. I was nervous and had my doubts but made a commitment and didn't want to let anyone down, including myself. My commitment was so strong to make the gastric bypass work and to be in the best possible health. I exercised to maintain strength in my legs since I knew I would have to walk a lot after the surgery to keep from getting pneumonia and to help heal. I even quit smoking and gave up coffee. My husband had doubts about the surgery, but was very supportive and willing to help me any way he could. He wanted me to be healthy but was concerned about me going through any surgery.

The intravenous (IV) needle was inserted into my arm and I was wheeled into the surgery room. I had been given some drugs to relax, but do remember saying, no. It was too late. When I awoke I remember my first words were, "Oh Damn". It really hurt; the nurses hooked me up to a morphine pump once I got into my room for the pain. I have never been in favor of using drugs, but at this point I was grateful I had that pump to control the pain. I was groggy, yet glad it was over. I was ready to begin the healing process. I didn't see Dr. No, who did my gastric bypass surgery, until my six week check-up. He had passed me off to one of his associates immediately following the surgery, left on vacation, and didn't call to check up on me. I had no complications while in the hospital and all seemed to be going well.

The first day I was home from the hospital I noticed two open sores on the right side of my body under my arm. I called up Dr. No's office and told the nurse about these sores and that they were very painful. The nurse told me to go to my family physician for help with these sores.

I went that day to my family doctor and was given a prescription for antibiotics. The antibiotics made me nauseous and I vomited for two days. After the protein shake I was trying to drink came up, I had dry heaves which was painful. I called my surgeons office again and was advised by an associate doctor to stop taking the antibiotics.

I was so weak from the vomiting and in pain, but was not advised to go to the hospital to get checked in case I broke the staple line and stitches. I was concerned the silastic ring could have moved from all the vomiting and dry heaves. This concern was dismissed by Dr. No's associate. I requested that I go to the hospital to get checked and was told I wasn't sick enough. The associate doctor told me to keep drinking water and try to get in the protein shakes.

Over the next several weeks I kept trying to get in fluids as instructed while waiting for my six week check-up to get help for the sores and to get answers about my inability to get the protein drinks down. I stayed in my recliner chair for those weeks since sleeping in bed was uncomfortable. After six weeks sleeping in that chair, I was about ready to have the thing tossed out the door.

During those long six weeks I tried to drink the protein shakes recommended by Dr. No, but I was continuously nauseous. Getting in protein drinks was a big problem; I became lactose intolerant so many proteins were incompatible with my system. Soy protein drinks made me ill as well, along with every other product available in the stores. I knew I needed protein to heal so I put up with the nausea to get in the nutrients. I was very determined to make this work and wouldn't give up trying to find protein I could keep down. I took the advice from Dr. No's nurse and nutritionist to keep trying other proteins and was told the nausea would go away with time, but it didn't. I either vomited, became nauseous or both from the day I came home from the hospital, and it continued every day for more than eighteen months.

The only pleasure I had at that time was my daily walks outside. Walking lifted my spirit in so many ways, and since I live in the country, I was able to feel the love of Mother Earth. I new I had to try something to bring some sense of joy in my life since trying to get in protein drinks was a daily struggle.

Even though my spirit was trying to bring my mind and body into a balance, it was not happening. I felt out of balance and struggled every day, trying to get small sips of liquid in and hoped the vomiting would stop. I continued to check in with Dr. No's office to let the nurse know of my problem with getting in protein. The nurse referred me to the nutritionist which I called several times for help over the next several weeks. I tried what she recommended, yet the problems continued.

The nutritionist had run out of solutions for me regarding protein drinks so I decided to try foods that were high in protein. When I ate chicken or beef it would get stuck at the site I had the silastic ring put on below my small new stomach. No matter how much I chewed my food it would eventually come back out. The opening was only the size of a dime for food to pass through. When food got stuck it was painful and I would eventually throw it up.

I tried fish and that worked a little better, but there was still a problem with vomiting and being nauseous every day. I tried protein bars, but the sugar content is very high and with hypoglycemia, it was not an option. Sugar free products were also out of the question because of my bad reaction to artificial sweeteners. The taste of eggs was so repulsive I ruled those out, except on an occasional basis where I would eat one anyways just to get in protein.

I spent hours at the grocery store checking out food labels and health food stores for items containing protein. The cost of trying out foods high in protein had been astronomical. I ended up throwing most of it out because it either made me vomit, nauseous, or tasted so bad I couldn't choke it down if I had to.

It was suggested to try baby food and I tried that but was not successful in keeping down most of it. The fruits gave me hypoglycemic reactions and the taste was so bad I wondered how babies ever ate it. I wasn't willing to give up my search for food I could eat, but it was getting frustrating and very time consuming.

At this point I would try to get in the water I needed and the small amount of food before my six week check up with Dr. No. I was still only getting in 150 to 200 calories a day; a quarter cup of pureed soup several times a day. I pureed most of what I ate and stayed with soup and crackers. Eating very small bites and chewing very well. It took over an hour to get in a quarter cup. At least I was getting in something but wasn't sure exactly how much because of the vomiting. It could have been less than the 150 to 200 calories.

It was an all day job to get in any amount of nutrients and tried to get up to 300 calories because I was getting weaker every day. In between the constant vomiting and nausea I tried to get in the soup and water. There wasn't enough energy in me to do any daily activities that I use to do. My husband did all the cooking, shopping, laundry, and cleaning on top of holding down a full time job. He was getting tired and I knew it, this made me feel useless.

4

Follow Up Doctors

Visits

Dr. No, like most doctors' who do the weight loss surgeries, requires his patients to have follow-up visits after having the surgery. The visits usually are at the six week date after the surgery and then at the 3, 6, 9, and 12 month period. These follow-up visits are to check weight loss and to discuss questions and concerns. There are a few doctors that will see their patient longer than a year but that is not the norm.

I have heard from some patients that their doctor only required them to have a sixth month check-up and again at one year. These check-ups were for blood work-ups and weight checks. A good doctor will require their patients to have frequent check-ups and for longer than a year.

Six Week Check Up

During my six week check-up I had a list of problems I wanted Dr. No to address, but he only gave me ten minutes. He checked out the sores on my side and said he didn't know what they were, but thought they could be shingles.

I had already gone to my family doctor where he informed me the sores weren't shingles, and that a topical antibiotic would be best since I was vomiting. My family doctor told me it would most likely take several weeks to heal and leave scaring. For the next two months I kept these painful sores clean, applied topical antibiotics, and covered to prevent further irritation.

I reported to the nurse and Dr. No during my six week check-up that I was still having problems with any solid food. Dairy products had been eliminated at this point to help with my nausea, but it only made a very little difference. I was now lactose intolerant, could not take in NutraSweet™ because it gave me migraine headaches, frequent vomiting, and I was allergic to all citric foods. I was also experiencing "dumping" several times a day, even though I was not consuming any sugar. Dumping happens when a person with the gastric bypass eats sugar. There is severe nausea, sweats, diarrhea, and lack of energy. Most often a person has to lie down because they feel so bad. My hair was falling out at an alarming rate and I went from sweating to being so cold I stayed in the shower a lot to get warm. My muscles hurt throughout my whole body. I was beginning to get depressed over this situation.

I know exercising helps with depression, and with a lack of energy I felt it important to try to get in some exercise other than short walks outside. The information in the literature Dr. No gave me emphasized exercising so we bought a treadmill which I started at a slow pace and short distance. I was looking forward to increasing my exercise program to include many of the activities I had done before the surgery. I told Dr. No I was increasing my exercising and he agreed that I should be as active as possible.

I later learned that exercise can help with depression, but when the body is in starvation, it can be more harmful than helpful. A body depleted of nutrients cannot keep going and will eventually shut down; the immune system will also be compromised. I wanted to exercise and get back to a normal life. Also, I knew I would have to get in more food in order to sustain the activity level I wanted.

I followed the food list given to me by Dr. No regarding what to eat and what to avoid. I had no energy and feeling emotionally spent from trying foods only to end up vomiting. The nausea was overwhelming, but again I was told by the nurse that this will soon go away along with the pain when I ate.

The entire six week check up lasted all of ten minutes and no advice given to help with getting in more protein, nor a remedy or reason for having chronic nausea and vomiting. I had already tried everything the nurse recommended regarding getting in protein. I was able to get in the water I needed, vitamins, calcium supplements, and B-12 tablets that melted under my tongue. I could not take any vitamins that had sugar or artificial sweeteners so I crushed up vitamins that did not have these in them and tried to get them down. It usually took about an hour to get in the recommended dose.

I was crying at Dr. No's office because I was exhausted from trying so hard to get in food and feeling so weak. I was originally told by Dr. No that I would have more energy after having the gastric bypass surgery, and the opposite was happening. I did not get any support or medical advice that would help me with my problems from Dr. No and his nurse. They told me to call people on the calling list to see if they could offer help. I thought this rather odd since I wanted medical advice and felt Dr. No should be giving me the help I was asking for.

I called Pat from the calling list since I spoke with her many times prior to the gastric bypass surgery and wanted to see if she could offer help. I was shocked! What she proceeded to tell me completely floored me and left me devastated. Pat told me she had several problems with her surgery, but didn't tell me because she wanted me to have the surgery. She said it changed her life and the problems were worth it since she could now fit into smaller clothes. Pat informed me she had problems with chronic vomiting and had two endoscope procedures to see if there was a problem The procedures didn't show there was anything wrong so she accepted the fact that she would probably always have problems with vomiting. It was alright with her, as long as she was able to wear smaller clothes.

Pat told me she smoked marijuana to alleviate the nausea and vomiting. Pat also told me the marijuana helped with the daily depression and it was her way to cope with life after her WLS (Weight Loss Surgery).

Pat also had numb feet and hands, but said it was still worth it all. After hearing about these problems, and others, I finally asked her why she just wasn't truthful with me in the beginning. Pat felt that I might change my mind and not have the surgery, which she felt was the best thing for me. I had trusted her and felt betrayed by her deception.

Even though I was hurt by Pat's deception I did talk with her a couple of times after the conversation where she admitted she was not truthful with me. I still had hoped that she could help me because I had no where else to turn. The end to our relationship came when she told me not to ever say anything but positive comments about the surgery. Being thin was more important to her than being healthy and she didn't want me to bring up problems again. Pat told me she would slap me across the face if I ever brought up any dissatisfaction with the gastric bypass surgery in the future. She advised me to say only good things to others so they too will have the surgery. I was stunned! She threatened me with bodily harm if I ever said anything negative about the gastric bypass surgery and from the tone in her voice I knew she meant it. This was a woman who was on the support call list given to me by Dr. No and I had once felt would be honest with me and supportive. I would no longer have any contact with Pat.

I also called two other people I had spoken with prior to the surgery to see if they could offer any advice. They both told me that I must not be following the diet plan correctly and it was most likely my fault things weren't working out for me. So much for any help!

Three Month Check Up

I reported to Dr. No and his nurse that I had increased my exercise to include an hour on the treadmill every day. It was a struggle to exercise since my energy level was not getting any better. I was living on about 300 calories per day since most of what I took in was coming back out. Dr. No advised me to increase my caloric intake, but I reminded him that I was trying yet the food would not stay in and the nausea had continued every day. Dr. No told me before I had the surgery I would not be hungry. I was hungry all the time yet, suffered with the nausea when I did. *It was easier not to eat* than to lie on the couch with nausea and the pain from eating. By not eating I was becoming weaker, but when I did eat, I was so ill. It was a dilemma I continuously had to deal with every hour of the day.

I was having a problem with uncontrollable shaking hands, fatigue, sweating, anxiety, craving of sweets even though I could not have sugar, lactose intolerant, headaches, being cold, dry skin and hair, muscle pain, confusion, and my vision was becoming blurred. I went to the optometrist for new glasses, but that did not help. I could read the small print on labels easier, but the blurred vision was still there along with headaches.

The headaches were something new to me; I have never had headaches on an every day basis and did not know the cause. Clarity of my mind was always an asset, but now it was disappearing and being replaced with confusion. I had already been in menopause for several years since having a complete hysterectomy and knew what it was like to have my mind wonder from time to time, but this was completely different. There were many days I couldn't remember if I took all my supplements. I started keeping a daily journal of what I took and when to keep track of everything I was taking. I didn't know if I was experiencing Alzheimer problems or just wasn't getting in enough food.

Depression was setting in due to a lack of food; my body was not getting in sufficient nutrients even though I was trying to get in everything Dr. No told me to do. I wasn't used to crying, but was doing so again in Dr. No's office. I kept asking for help, but was told it would get better and not to worry. He said to go home and eat more food and wasn't concerned about the fact that I had chronic vomiting and nausea.

I still was not able to eat any fruits, vegetables, bread, rice, and a host of other foods. It is easier to say what I could eat, which was broth or pureed soup than to try and list all the foods that I couldn't eat. I did work at getting in my water every day without vomiting. Hair loss was still a problem and I was just told to keep eating protein. I was struggling and did not know what to do. I told Dr. No I couldn't eat protein because solid food wouldn't stay down, no matter how much I chewed it but my concern was ignored. So, I would continue following the recommendation to exercise in hope that it all would get better. I would also keep trying to get down protein drinks even though they made me sick.

Dr. No implied my problems were all in my head and exercising would improve my disposition. He appeared to be more concerned with how much I lost rather than addressing my questions and concerns. My three month check-up lasted all of ten minutes and then I was dismissed.

Sixth Month Check Up

As usual, my time with Dr. No lasted no more than five to ten minutes at best. Again, the nurse and Dr. No seemed to be more interested in my weight loss than my health. My health had continued to deteriorate even though the blood tests showed I was in normal range, whatever that means. My caloric intake was still at 300 calories a day and not enough to sustain an exercise regime.

Dr. No told me exercise was vital to improved health and weight loss. Daily activity was something I enjoyed very much and wanted to continue. I had to reduce my exercise to an hour a day or less, and knew it was only a matter of time where that would be impossible for me to do. I began to lose control and fall down several times a day from muscle weakness, fatigue and dizziness. After an incident in the mountains I worried about my physical well being and if I could ever be able to go for a walk again.

The weather was beautiful so I decided to walk outside instead of using my treadmill. Living in the mountains is a wonderful place to get out and walk. I had gradually built up walking a distance of four miles a day in the months following my surgery. I couldn't do all four miles at once and sat down frequently to rest.

One day while I was out for a walk, my legs gave out on me and I fell down. My legs felt like noodles and I knew something was not right, but had no idea as to what the problem was. My car was two miles away and I was not sure how I was going to get there to drive home. Luckily, a man came by and asked if he could help me. This wonderful man took me back to my car and I was able to drive myself home. The rest of the day I had no energy and just sat in my chair. I kept trying to get in protein to enhance my energy. I decide to go out walking a couple of times a week instead of every day, but that didn't work either. I still kept falling down and needed assistance, so I made the decision to stop going out for walks all together. I knew I couldn't risk going out and not having help to get me home, even though I loved walking. This literally broke my heart to not go outside and see the wild rabbits running around, or watching the deer with their fawns playing. Getting in nutrients would have to be my main priority, exercising would have to be put on hold for the time being.

I continued trying to get in protein, vitamins, B-12, calcium and water, but they were not helping they way I was told they would. Hair loss was still a problem along with hand tremors. The nurse advised me to see a neurologist for the tremors and did not mention the problems I was having could be due to the surgery. I was concerned that my problems appeared to be dismissed so easily. I felt Dr. No and the nurse just wanted me to go away so they wouldn't have to deal with the condition I was in.

The nausea and vomiting continued every day and it was wearing me out. I was so cold all the time, and stayed wrapped up in a blanket most of the day. At night, I would not get any sleep as a result of the need to constantly take the blankets on and off. I would have sweats and be completely soaked, and would have to get up to change clothes. The sweats would be followed by freezing cold. I could not get enough blankets on me to stay warm. Often, I would get up and take a hot shower to get warm again. This occurred during the day as well, and was not what I had experienced the previous six years in menopause.

I also was having heart palpitations on a daily basis that I never had before the gastric bypass surgery. It scared me to have my heart race so fast and then skip beats. My breathing became labored. The rapid heart rate was followed by a slow down of my pulse to where I had no energy to walk across the room. The heart palpitations frequently occurred early in the morning before getting out of bed. I had mentioned this to Dr. No and his nurse but they didn't seem concerned with this problem.

In hindsight, I know I should have gone to the emergency room, but my thought process was distorted by the lack of food and depression. I wasn't thinking clearly and dismissed my husbands' suggestions to get help at the hospital. If all my problems were in my head like Dr. No thought, then I would look like a fool if I went to the emergency room. I kept thinking all these problems would go away soon and my body was just going through an adjustment to the surgery.

By six months I had also thought my scar from the gastric bypass surgery would finally stop hurting, but it had not. I still could not wear clothes that would touch the scar nor could I sleep on my stomach. Sleeping on my stomach would hurt and cause the nausea to become worse. I tried several ointments and lotions to try to alleviate the soreness but nothing worked.

I was advised by Dr. No to continue as I was doing and he would see me in three months. I was crying and wanted help, but he just did not seem to care at all. I left his office with no answers to my problems and felt so alone with this dilemma.

By this point I became more depressed than I ever thought possible. In thirty two years together, my husband had only seen me cry a few times and now he was watching helplessly as I broke down every day. On several occasions, I was so depressed with uncontrollable crying; my husband would take time off from work to come home to be with me.

I had always been a most happy person, despite being overweight. I loved life, and now the happiness was gone. I so wanted to be back to the way I was where I could do activities with my husband and children. My physical and mental health had deteriorated to the point that I could not do any activities. My life had not improved for the better, but rather went further downhill.

Dr. No s' concern seemed more about how much I had lost in weight rather than my well being. He told me I should be down another thirty pounds by my next office visit which was in three months.

I felt he might be in a rush to go to another patient, because in the middle of my questions to him he just got up and walked out the door. He leaned his head back in though the doorway and said he would see me in three months.

I went home disappointed with my sixth month visit with Dr. No, but also felt I would try to increase my caloric intake as recommended to see if I would feel better.

During the next three weeks I tried to take in very small amounts of food every waking hour. Solid food came right back out so I stayed mainly with pureed soup and other foods that I could put in the blender. I never thought this would be so time-consuming and challenging, but I did it.

I had been keeping a weekly log of my weight loss along with my journal, but decided to put the scales away for the entire three weeks. Scales are not a good idea to keep around, and the reason I weighed once a week was to put it on the log sheet provided by Dr. No.

I had been keeping a log of the amount of calories I had been taking in on a daily basis and never realized how hard it would be to get in more than 300 to 500 calories a day. With the 500 daily calorie intake I had been able to maintain my weight, not gaining or losing. The more food I tried getting in the sicker I became.

Still, the 500 calories a day I was trying to get in was not enough for me to continue exercising. I increased my intake to 600 calories per day and was struggling with the nausea even more than before, but tried to push through it. I pureed soup and drank it all day to try to get in more calories. The soup was going through my system so fast that there wasn't any way the nutrients were going to be absorbed.

By the end of the three week period I had not felt any better at 600 calories a day. I decided to weigh myself to see if I was still maintaining my weight. I had gained fifteen pounds in that three week period on 600 calories a day. I couldn't understand how I could gain weight when the soup was passing through my system so fast. I talked with the nurse at Dr. No's office about the weight gain and she said I should not have gained but to keep eating and the gaining would stop and I would begin losing again.

For the next two weeks I had stayed at 600 calories a day and still was not losing weight or feeling better. I was not concerned with the weight gain; I was concerned with the lack of improved health. I called Dr. No's office and told the nurse about the weight gain and that I was still not feeling better. I told her that I had been following everything they had told me to do, and that the nausea had gone on way too long. I asked her if I should go back down in calories and she said, "I probably would if I were you", so I did. Trying to increase my calorie intake to 600 calories a day was a disaster. I was vomiting so much I couldn't leave the house to take a walk. I kept my 'barf bowl' with me at all times because I couldn't always make it to the kitchen sink or to the bathroom. When I wasn't vomiting I stayed either in bed or on the couch from being so nauseous.

I went back down to 500 calories a day and felt a little better because eating made me nauseous. After a week at 500 calories a day I went back down to 300. Food was making me sick, and the less I ate the less I felt nauseous and the less I vomited. I gradually lost the weight I had gained while getting in more calories. After awhile I was back to maintaining my weight on 300 calories a day and after a few weeks lost a few more pounds. I could have cared less if lost anymore weight. It wasn't worth it if I had to live a life of misery and pain.

The big question I had, which Dr. No could not answer was; would I have to stay at 500 calories a day the rest of my life to maintain my weight. Dr. No initially told me I would be able to eat 1,000 to 1,500 calories a day once I lost the weight I needed, according to his charts.

Before the surgery I ate 300 calories a day to lose and maintained my weight at 500 calories. I was now no better off than before I had the gastric bypass surgery when it came to the amount of food I could eat, except now I was nauseous most of the time and struggled with vomiting.

It would have been easier and healthier if my husband locked me in a room with a treadmill and had passed an apple and a small piece of skinless chicken to me once a day until I lost weight. I can't say I would have been happy with him for doing this to me and probably would have wanted to do bodily harm to him, but at least I wouldn't have been vomiting and nauseous. I would still have the same weight loss as having the gastric bypass surgery but without the damage done to my body from the surgery.

One of the reasons I decided to have the gastric bypass surgery in the first place was because I did not want to go down in calories again like I did on my own before. I did not feel good then and did not feel good now. At least before the surgery, I could eat more without getting nauseous and did not have bouts of vomiting several times a day. I could also do some exercising without ending up on the ground from weakness.

The constant falling left bruises that took a long time to heal. I also was able to absorb nutrients before the surgery where it was not occurring after the gastric bypass.

The information in the literature provided by Dr. No had stated weight loss was permanent. I asked Dr. No about this and after skirting the issue for several minutes he did say, "Some gained back the weight they lost but if they did they were failures".

I have talked with patients who have had the RNY gastric bypass surgery who said they have gained weight back, but that they can always go back to induced vomiting to get their weight back down. This is not only unhealthy from a nutritional stand point but also hard on the staple line inside where the stomach has been altered. Chronic vomiting can also cause problems with the esophagus, heart, stomach, and teeth. The vomiting can also cause the pouch to burst which worried me a great deal.

I do not know the statistics regarding how often the pouch bursts. It is best to ask your doctor about the probability of this happening. A woman told me her pouch burst when she ate too much and vomited many times a day. Bulimics have many physical problems and I didn't go into this surgery with the intent of becoming a bulimic or anorexic.

I decided it was best to try to get in 300 calories a day and vomit less than to try to get in more pureed soup and vomit all day long. I would try to get more rest and wait for my nine month check up.

Nine Month Check Up

My health continued to deteriorate and my visit with Dr. No had not been any more helpful than the last few office visits.

I was having heart palpitations on a daily basis and did not know why, and it scared me since my father died of heart failure.

I was still falling down when I took short walks and was dizzy, no matter how much protein, vitamins, minerals, water, and calcium I took in. I was also falling down in my home and when I went out shopping. Several times I would just sit down on the floor in the grocery store or bookstore so I would not end up on the ground and risk hurting myself. I told Dr. No about this and he told me to reduce my exercise since I was not getting in enough food to sustain my activity level. He also told me to just go home and eat.

I was crying at this point out of frustration and despair. I could not understand how he could say "just eat more" when I told him I was vomiting eight times a day and sometimes more and was continuously nauseous.

Dr. No felt, according to my medical records, my emotions had become volatile because of the crying and recommended I go to my family physician for further help. I asked him if he thought I might need hormone replacement therapy to help with the depression. Again, he told me to go to another doctor for help, explaining that he did not handle those problems.

I did go to my family physician and gynecologist for help as recommended by Dr. No. Both said they would work with me, but felt Dr. No should have been more involved with my health matters. They also felt I should talk with Dr. No about having the reversal of the gastric bypass to eliminate the problems I had on an ongoing basis.

My husband accompanied me on my nine month visit with Dr. No. He was there to help me in case I collapsed due to muscle fatigue and weakness, and to talk with Dr. No about having the gastric bypass surgery reversed. I had many questions about the procedure and what it entailed. As I started to talk with Dr. No about the reversal he stopped me in the middle of a question and looked me straight in the eyes and said, "*If you think I am going to reverse this surgery you better get that out of your head right now. It will not be done.*"

I tried to remind him of his original statement about reversing the gastric bypass surgery if there were any health problems with it. He did not want to even address the question and walked out of the office.

As we sat there for a moment in his office we both looked at each other and felt such a feeling of despair. Dr No had turned down what seemed to be the only solution to my problems. He had not given me any other solutions and I was becoming weaker by the day and more despondent.

I walked out of his office and never wanted to go back to him again. I felt that I had been deserted by Dr. No when I had believed he would be there for me.

My husband and I went home feeling lost with nowhere to go for help. We both knew at that point Dr. No wasn't going to help me. I am not a quitter and tried hard to push through all the problems. I followed every thing in Dr. No's booklet and what he and his nurse recommended.

If I had not eaten very slowly, had fluids with my meals, ate sugar, and all the other things that as patients we were told not to do, and then I could see why some of the problems would occur. This was not the case; I was an excellent patient and had a determination to follow all the rules for a healthy life with the gastric bypass surgery.

Ten Month Doctor's Visit

At ten months out from my gastric bypass surgery I went back to Dr. No's office, but this time I saw Dr. No's associate.

I had placed a call into the office the night before and told the associate that I was having a lot of problems, and feeling so weak that I could not walk any distance without falling down.

Dr. No's associate said as long as I was getting in water I could not be admitted to the hospital and given an IV to replenish fluids. If my condition became worse he would do this, but felt by coming in and talking with him the next day he would clarify my questions and concerns.

I also went in to see him because I could not stop crying and was at the end of my rope and tired of going through this any more. My husband was with me and we wanted to discuss having the gastric bypass reversed.

This new doctor sat with us for an hour reviewing my history since having the surgery. He told us that a reversal was not a problem if that is what I wanted.

We told him that Dr. No had already refused to even discuss this option. The doctor told us it was up to Dr. No to make the decision since he would be the one that would do the reversal.

My husband and I returned home and discussed our options. I could stay the way I was or look for another doctor. I would begin looking for a doctor to help me with my physical problems or to get the gastric bypass reversed if Dr. No's office gave up on me completely. I didn't want to have to resort to this measure, but my options were diminishing every month that went by.

I was not willing to sit back and slowly die without doing everything I could to get better. My depression was getting the best of me and that made me even more dejected.

I want to note that during the first 10 months I had lost 120 pounds and was unhappy. The unhappiness had nothing to do with adjusting to the loss of weight but rather that I was in worse health than I had ever been. For me, it wasn't worth all that I had to go through and continued to endure. During the next 8 months I had lost 10 pounds even though I still only consumed 300 calories a day and sometimes up to 500. My body found its set point and weight loss stopped. From what I have learned from others, this is quite common.

Eleven Month Doctor's Visit

After eleven months of nausea, vomiting, depression, weakness, fatigue and other difficulties I went back to Dr. No's associate for help.

I was finally given Compazine® to help with the nausea which I tried for a month, but it did very little. I discontinued taking Compazine® when Dr. No's office did not want to refill the prescription.

I didn't want to battle over this and didn't have the strength to fight them. I was already taking so many pills (vitamins and supplements), and didn't want to live the rest of my life on more, especially since I would have to increase the dosage of Compazine® to get any relief. There was no guarantee this medication would alleviate the nausea.

The side effects from the drug also played an important decision in not wanting to take more than I had to. I wanted to be off of drugs, not to increase medications to get through the day. I didn't want to take drugs that masked my problems; I wanted solutions to my problems.

At this point it was hard to eat and keep down a cup of soup per day along with all the medications. I was trying to get in 300 calories a day, but had to settle with what I could. There were many days I didn't have a thing to eat, it just wasn't worth the effort. My lab tests showed I was in the normal range which was not that surprising after reading about malnutrition.

I later learned through reading medical literature, and talking with the naturopath, that it can take a long time before the tests will reveal what is going on in the body. The naturopath I went to told me blood tests can show everything is fine and in normal range, but they don't always tell what is the long term damage being done to the body.

The eleven month visit to Dr. No's office was my last one. The associate doctor was sending me back to Dr. No for future weight check ups. I wasn't getting the answers I was looking from Dr No, so I saw no reason to go back to him.

Dr. No's associate also told me to go to my family physician with any further problems regarding depression. Again, I was left out in the cold without help. I never heard from Dr. No or his nurse again for any follow up, even when they knew I was not doing well. As far as they were concerned, my surgery was a success and the problems I was having were all in my head.

5

The Breakdown

One morning I woke up and tried to feed the dogs and work up enough energy to start my daily activities. By this point, my activities consisted of putting out food and water for the birds, cleaning the kitchen and taking care of the dog's food and water. Instead of doing these routine tasks I ended up on the living room floor in a heap crying uncontrollably.

I was having a complete breakdown and my world as I knew it was crumbling. My husband stayed with me even though he was needed at work for an important meeting. He felt I was more important and could not be left alone. Never in my life have I asked for help, and now I was in no position to refuse it.

I did not know what was causing my depression, but I gathered up enough strength to call my gynecologist to get an appointment for hormone replacement therapy. I didn't know what else it could be. Before the gastric bypass surgery I had some mood swings, but this was way over the top. It was not who I normally was.

I saw the gynecologist and was put on hormones and was told they would not take effect for a few weeks. I did not have a few weeks to wait for them to kick in. I decided to take them anyway and hope they would work on me sooner rather than later.

Two weeks had gone by and still no improvement with my severe depression. For someone like me who never had depression in their life it was devastating.

It was also depressing having to eliminate more foods from my diet. I had become allergic to wheat products as well as all citric foods, fruits and juices, vegetables, rice, and all dairy products. Leaving out fried foods was not a problem since I never ate that kind of food anyway, and rarely drank alcohol or sodas. There was not much else to eat so I drank broth.

The increasing number of problems I was experiencing had finally taken a toll on my mental health. I cried most of the day and did not know why, or how to stop it. I knew I needed help, and so I decided to go to my family physician.

My family doctor had originally recommended the gastric bypass for me because I qualified by being over 100 pounds overweight. I saw him nine months after having the surgery and he became concerned about my health. After examining me he said, "He would no longer recommend the surgery to his patients." *He felt I had maybe one to five years to live if I kept the gastric bypass in place.*

I wasn't the first patient of his who had problems after the surgery. He had been led to believe, by the information he had obtained regarding the gastric bypass surgery that it was safer than what he was now seeing in his patients.

Although, I didn't want to change doctors, I now had to look for another family doctor because the company my husband works for changed insurance plans.

I found a new family physician the same month I left my previous family doctor. I will call my new doctor, Dr. Caring, because that is the kind of doctor she is. She sat with me for about an hour to go over my medical records from Dr. No. Dr. Caring ran tests and gave me an exam, something I was not used to from Dr. No, and realized this is what I had needed all along. She did not just look at me hoping I would go away; rather she took a real caring attitude regarding my entire health.

Dr. Caring finally came up with my diagnosis and it was a relief to know what the problem was. The problem wasn't in my head, but in my body! I was suffering from malnutrition from having the gastric bypass surgery. The shaking of my hands was due to hypoglycemia.

Dr. Caring was able to diagnose the hypoglycemia problem on my first visit with her. I wanted to know about hypoglycemia so I bought a book to read up on it. Getting information on this condition was most important to me and I wanted to be armed with all the knowledge I could get to understand hypoglycemia.

The symptoms of hypoglycemia are numerous, but there are a few that can trigger further testing to confirm the diagnosis. It's important to have your doctor run tests before diagnosing hypoglycemia to confirm whether you might have this problem or not. Some of the problems are: dizziness, blurred vision, depression, anxiety, crave sweets, fatigue, headache if meals skipped, sleepy after meals, cry easily and confused, unexplained sweating, insomnia, fainting spells, irritability, and more.

I had all these symptoms and yet Dr. No did not pick up on this easily diagnosed problem, nor did he give me a blood test to determine the cause of some of my problems.

Some people who had the gastric bypass surgery that I spoke with told me they could tolerate only a small amount of sugar and others like me could not handle even the smallest amount. I couldn't tolerate NutraSweet® at all so avoiding sugar was very important. I was already following a sugar free diet and still could not understand why I was having hypoglycemia.

When I understood that skipping meals could trigger this condition I tried to eat more often. The problem was keeping the food in and dealing with the nausea. The protein drinks had sugar in them as well so I was left with drinking broth. I found out quickly that broth did not have enough nutrients in it to sustain a healthy life.

The problems with hair loss, numbness in my toes, weakness, memory loss, heart palpitations, muscle failure, pain in my muscles and bones, and continued crying was due to lack of nutrients. I was not absorbing nutrients from the food or vitamins I was taking, even though I had more than doubled up on the amount of supplements. I had wondered at this point how much permanent damage had been done to my body as a result of my surgery. It concerned me, but finally felt I was now getting the medical attention I needed to improve my health.

I was also given medication for under active thyroid. Thyroid problems run in my family and half of them were already on medication to treat this problem, even though the numbers from my blood tests did not show there was a problem. Dr. Caring told me that numbers do not always reveal a problem with the thyroid. I had every one of the symptoms of a thyroid problem and it was worth a try to see if I felt better. After only a short time on the medication for thyroid, several of my symptoms lessened.

I recalled that I told Dr. No during the initial consultation office visit that there might be a problem with my thyroid and should that be addressed prior to the surgery. He gave me a look of disgust and said he did not think that was my problem and dismissed my concerns. Looking back, I feel that if only he would have taken me seriously all of this might have been corrected without surgery.

According to Dr. Caring, thyroid problems can occur after the gastric bypass surgery and if you had this as an existing problem it could become much worse after the surgery. It takes a caring and qualified doctor to keep a close watch on you so you don't get into further trouble with a thyroid imbalance.

In addition to thyroid medication, I was put on Celexa® for chemical depression. It would take a few weeks before the medication for depression would take effect, and this had me concerned since I was having trouble getting through the day by myself. I was started off on very low doses of Celexa® so it would not cause more nausea than I already had.

My husband could no longer take any more time off from work and yet I could not handle life alone. This was just not who I was before all of this started. I use to enjoy hours and days alone in meditation and now I could not be left alone for a few minutes. I had hit rock bottom and could not handle life any longer. I also gave up eating unless my husband made me drink the pureed soup. I just could not stand throwing up anymore and was exhausted from the chronic nausea. It just was not worth the effort and I didn't have the energy to put up a fight by myself.

Dr. Caring put me on Xanax® for anxiety to help me through the days and nights until the antidepressant took effect. This was a relief for me to finally get some help, but I still had a long way to go and my husband did not feel I should be left alone. He offered to pay airfare to my twin sister, Danica, so that I would have help and she accepted.

Danica and I are very close and she knew something was wrong with me (see Danica's letter in Chapter 9 - Family and Friends Support). She was the only one I had told about the surgery, and to honor my privacy she kept it quiet from the rest of the family. This was my choice and when I was ready I would let the rest of them know about the surgery and what I had been going through.

There wasn't any shame in having a gastric bypass nor did I feel like a failure because I resorted to this procedure. I have always kept my personal life private and didn't feel at that time they could be of any help. I was wrong in that belief and later would find them to be more supportive than I ever thought possible. For people like me who are very self-reliant, asking for help is not easy, but eventually it needs to be embraced.

Asking for Danica's help saved my life, and if it weren't for her staying with me for two weeks I probably would not be here today. The thought of taking my life was overwhelming. I just wanted the problems to end and felt like I was at the bottom of the barrel with no way out. I had all the pills in my hand and a glass of water. Then I realized that even if I had tried to swallow pills to end my life, it wouldn't have worked. They would just be vomited up anyways so why even try. I didn't know whether to cry or laugh at the situation. Besides, I had a strong will to get my health back and made a decision to fight for my life. My sorrow subsided and was replaced with an inner strength to get back control over my life.

There had to be a way out of the bottom of that barrel and I was going to do all that I could to climb out. I have never been a quitter in my life, and I wasn't about to give into feelings of ending it when I had so much to live for. My children, husband, family, and friends were too important to me to leave this life by my own hands. It was at this point in my life that I decided, "**I Want To Live!**" I also knew I needed therapy to get me clear on the decisions I had to make for my future.

Danica came with me to my therapy session, and she reminded me I had a lot to live for and that my work here on Mother Earth was not over and that the future included the joy I once had.

Danica also made sure I ate frequently to get in the nourishment my body needed to get my health back. I know it was hard for her to see me sit and cry for hours and struggle to get in food. She had never seen me this way before. It saddened my heart to ask for so much help and not be the strong person I had once been. Deep down I knew the strength was still inside of me and I would get it back.

When in complete despair, it is difficult, but not impossible to see the way back to a balanced life by taking one step at a time. I needed help with that first step and then the next would come and prepare me for the rest of the steps. With each passing moment there is a chance to change the outcome of the future. I was ready to take the steps to change the future of my life.

At the same time I was working on taking these steps to improvement my mind, body, and spirit I had another obstacle to overcome. I was no longer able to keep my business going and had to give it up. It had brought me so much joy that it was devastating to have to put it aside for now.

At this point in my life I had lost so much; my health, my business, and a quality of life I was told would be improved by having the gastric bypass surgery.

I plan to restart my business at some point, but need to concentrate on my health first and the rest will come when the time is right. I was just not able at that time to get the energy and physical strength I needed to continue working.

I needed to prioritize my life and to put in order what was important first, which was my health, and then go on from there. It's not selfish to put ones self first when it comes to being healthy. Caregivers tend to take care of others first and themselves last. This belief had to change and I was willing to try therapy to resolve this pattern I had set for myself.

My family was happy that I finally decided to take care of me and they supported my choice to seek help. They wanted me to be happy again and have my life back, one day at a time.

6

Therapy

I started going to a therapist and the same time I was put on anti-depressants. The anti-depressants would take awhile to make any difference with my mental state, and I believe you cannot just take medication by itself without therapy. Medication is a tool to help you be able to get to a point where you can work on problems. My problem was getting my health back, and how I was going to do that.

According to Dr. Caring, my family doctor, there was a chemical imbalance in my body that left me struggling to get control of my life. If you have to struggle with anything, then you are out of balance.

This does not just have to do with physical problems, but everything else as well. I have always strived for balance and was determined to get it back no matter how much work there is to do. I see work as an opportunity to grow and gain strength with all aspects of life. I was ready and willing to do what I needed to do to get back control of my own destiny.

My first therapist was good, but she was not going to be covered by my insurance plan. She referred me to another therapist after a few weeks of working with her.

The second therapist and I bonded immediately. She is wonderful! She did not give me sympathy, which I liked. She did give me empathy which allowed me to reach out and take control over my life. I will call her Dr. Healer since she helped me remember how I can heal my mind, body, and spirit. I have the tools to heal myself; they just got misplaced for awhile when all my energy went towards sustaining my physical body.

Dr. Healer was with me every step of the way as I went forward in getting my life back. Tools such as therapy help open the doors so you can step through and do the work to find the answers to questions. Asking for help is not a weakness; it takes strength to want to be well. It takes courage to step up and say to yourself, I want to be healthier in all aspects of life, and help is there if you just take that first step. Help can be in the form of a therapist, family member, or friend. Once I put out my hand for help, I found others that would take it and walk with me as I continued on my journey to wellness.

I knew my health would improve once I got back the ability to absorb nutrients again. Dr. Healer helped me deal with the problems I had as a result of the chemical imbalance within my body. She had also helped me deal with the betrayal I experienced from Pat who deliberately deceived me about the problems she had by covering them up so I would have the gastric bypass surgery. There was also the feeling of betrayal from Dr. No and what I felt was his lack of compassion for my pain.

Betrayal is not new to me since it happened often in my life as a child. I was abused by those who professed to care about me, and took years of searching within to come to terms with the violations of myself and my sisters.

I do not regret anything that had happened to me as a child; it made me who I am today. I have more strength from living through adversity and keep moving forward. Learning from the past enabled me to take steps necessary to take back control of my life. I have been able to use this experience to help other children get through tough times. I am a person that will open my heart and arms to embrace anyone in need. It is healing for myself as well and has given me the opportunity to use the gifts I have to help others.

Dr. Healer's gift to me was being apart of my support team and preparing me for the gastric bypass reversal. She helped me "pack" for the surgery.

Packing included bringing together my mind, body, and spirit to a place where I am at ease with the choices I have made. I was becoming at peace within myself and I was bringing with me those people and items that gave me comfort and support.

Even though Dr. Healer couldn't be with me during my reversal surgery, I knew she would be with me in her heart. I was able to call her day or night. She was there for me before the reversal and after the surgery. Dr. Healer is truly a wonderful therapist and woman. I will always be grateful for her help during a difficult time in my life. I wish everyone in need could find a therapist like Dr. Healer. It makes a tremendous difference to have the support you deserve to move through any obstacle. I am grateful I had the best therapist that worked with me.

7

Naturopath

I will call the naturopath "Dr. Gentle" because of his approach to health care. I believe in alternative medicine and it seemed logical to see a specialist in an area where it is not intrusive and works with the balancing the body chemistry. I began seeing Dr. Gentle after being put on hormone replacement therapy and anti-depressants. I was still at the stage of crying most of the time and could not control my emotions.

My first appointment with Dr. Gentle consisted of giving him a complete rundown of my medical history, especially with the gastric bypass surgery. None of his prior patients had the surgery so it was new territory for him. Every naturopath has their own way of evaluating patients for imbalances in the body. At this point, I was willing to try this method, and to leave no door unopened in my search for improving my health.

In order for Dr. Gentle to have a complete understanding of the gastric bypass surgery he asked me to get my records from Dr. No. I called that day to get the records and was told to wait a few days before coming by the office to pick them up. When I first went to Dr. No, I had my medical records from my family physician sent to his office.

That evening I began reading all my records Dr. No's office gave me, including the ones sent to them from the family physician. Page by page I reviewed the information. I did not understand some of the terminology and what the blood tests meant, so I called a good friend of mine that is a nurse with many years of experience.

I will call this friend "Sunshine" since she has been a ray of hope and a wealth of knowledge that has been invaluable to me. Sunshine supported me throughout all phases of my experience with the gastric bypass. She was my nurse who took care of me while I recovered after surgery in the hospital. Sunshine was able to explain my records in detail and afterwards I was concerned about what I had found. I discovered errors in my medical records from Dr No's office, including the listing of a drug for hypertension for which I had never had a prescription.

To see a drug I had never taken on my medical records disturbed me a great deal.

So many things were running through my mind from these medical record findings. I felt concerned about these errors. Was this merely an oversight or something else happening? Were these inaccurate records used to get insurance approval? Many things ran through my mind for which there were no answers.

After looking back at the way I approached this surgery I could not find anything I did wrong before deciding to have the procedure. I went to the support group, talked with people on the support group call list given by Dr. No's office, had a consultation with Dr. No, read all the information provided by his office, and went on the internet to research the procedure.

I was devastated, but also knew that I had to move forward and could not put more energy into the past. It was over with and it was more important for me to concentration on getting better, physically as well as mentally.

I brought all this information and records into Dr. Gentle to evaluate before deciding on what I would need to improve my health.

Dr. Gentle's testing showed that all of my organs were under stress. They were not functioning in the normal range and that the blood tests taken before would not necessarily reveal what was actually happening in my body.

Dr. Gentle stated that since our bodies can only get simple carbohydrates from fat, it will draw nutrients and protein it needs, from organs and stored reserves to accommodate the blood tests. When calories are reduced to lose weight the first to go is the muscles, then the bones, and finally the fat!

Also, when reducing calories your body will think you are starving and will begin to store the smallest amount of nutrients, and weight loss will stop. The body can only do this for so long before physical problems become evident. Organs can start failing as well as the development of osteoporosis.

Osteoporosis can be a problem with the gastric bypass surgery and should not to be taken lightly. It is extremely painful – the individual feels a strong pain in their bones and as the disease progresses, the person can shatter bones very easily. For example; a person with osteoporosis can roll over in bed and break a rib. Individuals with osteoporosis are usually given strong narcotics like Morphine and even that does not take away the pain. Also osteoporosis can be very disabling.

Increasing the amount of exercise would help the muscles and bones, but in my case the malnutrition did not allow me to exercise. Vomiting and nausea prevented me from getting in the nutrients I needed to strengthen my body through exercise. I needed to eat more, but could not get it in to exercise more. Hopefully, Dr. Gentle would be able to give me supplements that will help with my absorption.

After Dr. Gentle completed his testing, he gave me tinctures, vitamins, minerals, and liquid calcium. The over the counter products I had been taking were not being absorbed. The ones Dr. Gentle recommended were designed to be more absorbent.

I also started on a rice protein with almond milk which worked for awhile. After a short time, the small amount of sugar in it started to put me back into hypoglycemia. The naturopath decided that being nauseous on the protein drinks was not a good idea so I went back to getting in protein through food.

I stayed with some fish and pureed soups, but it still did not provide the protein I needed. I was doing the best I could with what I had available, and that was all I could do under the circumstances.

Naturopaths can only do so much when the body has been altered. The organs work in unison with each other, so when the stomach is rearranged the other organs will be affected. Taking away the ability to absorb by bypassing the bottom part of the stomach puts undue stress on every organ in the body.

The naturopath was able to help me maintain by the supplements he gave me but there was no way of telling how long that would last. At least I was trying a way that would offer some kind of help.

I recommend going to a naturopath before having the gastric bypass surgery for help with obesity and related problems. Often times, a naturopath can find if there is an imbalance in the system which could cause weight gain.

By going to a naturopath weight loss might not be as fast as having the gastric bypass surgery, but it will have long lasting results with a higher level of physical well being.

I decided to continue going to Dr. Gentle since his treatment had been able to reduce some of the stress on my organs. The physical weakness, fatigue, nauseous feeling, dizziness, hypoglycemia, and depression had not been eliminated, but it seemed to improve somewhat. Dr Gentle stated he would find me a natural hormone replacement therapy I can take.

Testing still showed my organs were under stress and could start failing from the malnutrition and lack of absorption. Dr. Gentle is not pro-surgery, but felt at this point the reversal was needed for me to have a quality life. He would work with me to get as strong as possible to undergo the gastric bypass reversal and would continue working with me after the surgery.

8

Support Groups

I encountered many people who regret having the gastric bypass surgery, have had physical problems, wished they were more informed before the surgery, and had hoped to get better support.

I wondered how many people out there shared these same concerns and knew of others that are silently suffering. I have been asked why aren't these people going to their support group provided by their doctor and the answer is simple. They do not fit into what I call the, "cheerleading" group.

Many of us are very private people and do not feel comfortable sharing personal issues, physical as well as emotional, in front of a large group. Most of the people I spoke with that did not like their support group; felt many of the people going to them were advocates for WLS. While there were those that cried tears of joy over their weight loss, there were also those that cried tears of sorrow over their pain and suffering.

Not all support groups are this way and I feel many of these groups can be very helpful and encourage them to continue providing support. If you are lucky and have a good group, lead by a great doctor, then I say go for it. Otherwise, there are a lot of us who are shut down by the group if we bring up anything that sounds like we are dissatisfied with the outcome of our gastric bypass surgery. Some on-line support groups will remove you from the list if you bring up any negative side affects of the WLS.

In my case, Dr. No showed up for the support group meetings and answered questions. He never elaborated on the questions, giving a sentence or two and that was it.

Many of the questions asked in the support group should be answered during visits in his office where they can be directed to the patient and covered until the patient is satisfied. Dr. No gave me all of five minutes, and once gave me ten minutes to answer questions and left before I was through. There was not a chance to get answers to questions and when I did they were not adequate. He was in a hurry and had to get on to his next patient so I was suppose to wait until the next three month check up or go to the support group call list. Naturally, the people on the call list had the same problem, so they would have to improvise or fabricate answers for the potential new patient.

Support groups should not be expected to answer medical problems, the doctor should. Now that I am going to Dr. Compassion, the doctor who did my gastric bypass reversal, I am so glad to be given the time to have all my questions answered before I leave his office. This is how it should be and I praise those doctors that are providing the same kind of treatment. Unfortunately, this is not happening enough.

The support group I went to seemed to be more concerned with weight loss than overall health. Everyone went around the room saying their name and how much they lost. When I was leaving I heard two women talking how they must have failed because they had not lost as much weight as others in the group.

There were those that stated their health improved and they no longer had to take medication for diabetes and high blood pressure. I was happy they were having a positive experience with their gastric bypass, but what about the rest of those who were not healthy or happy with the procedure? I did not feel comfortable speaking up and saying, hey, I really do not like what I am going through, so I kept quiet. Nor did I feel like airing my problems for others to scrutinize.

Many people have written me stated they were very unhappy with their support group and would never go back. There are also letters from people considering the surgery who feel some of the support groups were more like revival meetings. Hyping people up and making them feel guilty and full of fear if they didn't have the surgery. Of course, they hear only from the people having a good experience and a few who did speak up about problems were quickly put down or the subject was changed. Like I said before, not all support groups are this way but there are many who infer the surgery is without complications. All sides should be discussed openly and honestly so people will have the whole story and not just the good ones. I hear from people often that the support group they attended didn't even bring up any stories about the downside of the surgery, only the good.

Another form of support is chat rooms for those who have had the gastric bypass surgery and for those considering it. I checked out these on-line sights several times and each time I went away more frustrated.

For the first few visits to an on-line site I just read what was being written to see what was being discussed. Those waiting for their surgery date to come would get all kinds of encouragement and how much better their life would be. They were repeatedly told how they would be able to wear smaller clothes and look great. Some wrote about physical problems and were given all kinds of advice. This kind of advice should be given by a *qualified doctor*, not a support group. I called this group the, "cheerleading" group since they sounded like a group of enthusiasts, similar to Dr. No's support group.

One day, I got up enough nerve to reveal that I was considering having the gastric bypass reversed, but that I was still looking into it and wanted more information. I thought maybe someone in the group might know of a web sight I could check out or put me in touch with others that already had theirs reversed.

The response I got from the support group on this web site when I mentioned reversal was more than I expected. I was berated like I never knew possible.

When I mentioned that in England they reverse all of the RNY procedures at a particular hospital, I was called a liar. I explained that I had checked it out thoroughly but they would not believe me. I was called crazy, weak willed, neurotic, a failure, an instigator, and more.

The group insisted that I give personal information about myself over the internet, and when I refused they accused me of making it all up. I noticed many of these people in this chat room had no problem telling the most intimate details about their personal lives, but I am not that way and shouldn't be expected to. I was asking specific questions and hoped I would get some answers from this support group. I did answer a few questions about my poor health and was blamed for not following what I was supposed to be doing. They said it was my fault that I was sick.

Another person I know, whose WLS was reversed told me she was treated the same way when she revealed she was going to have a reversal. She left the on-line support group in tears and would never go back. I have received many letters from people with problems that were treated in a very disrespectful manner. It isn't surprising that people looking into having the surgery get the impression everyone is happy with their WLS. If you are already having physical and emotional problems caused by the surgery why would you want further punishment from those who would rather attack you than to help you?

I also asked the on-line group what they knew about gaining back the weight. I had checked this out on the internet and found sixty percent of patients on average gained most, if not all, of it back after the five years. This number could be even higher since doctors are reluctant to publish long term weight loss statistics. Long term patients are also not followed for years after having the surgery so data is hard to come by.

When I asked the on-line group about the weight gain after the WLS many replied with, "Anyone who gains weight back is a failure." I can't understand how people in a support group with weight problems could call anyone a failure. Anyone who has had to deal with the treatment by a society that can't accept overweight people know how hurtful negative comments can be. A support group is designed to be understanding and have compassion for those that have endured the same kinds of problems.

I was not getting support, but, rather a heavy dose of attacking in this chat room. Many of those in the chat room told me to be quiet if I was not going to say positive things about the gastric bypass surgery because I might scare someone from having it by my questions. The questions I raised are important along with the other questions about problems people have so someone looking into the surgery knows what does happen to many people. Not everyone is going to have a great experience and everyone needs to be prepared in the event they have complications.

While in the chat room, I got messages on the side that the others could not read. They call this "whispering" in the chat room. Several were thanking me for bringing up the issue of a reversal and felt this should be brought up for discussion. They also had questions about the reversal and questions regarding where they could go for more information. Like myself, they wanted to draw on the wealth of experiences and knowledge from all those on-line to help direct them to resources available. They were very leery about bringing up anything that wasn't going to be received well by the group so kept it to themselves, especially since anyone who does isn't treated with respect.

The moderator apologized to me about how I was being treated and offered her phone number for me to call her if I wanted to have a personal conversation. I appreciated her concern and thanked her. I was not angry with the treatment received in the chat rooms, just sad. I thought the support group was about helping out all people. But, I was mistaken. I did not ask questions to upset anyone. Still, I wanted some answers or to be directed to a source where I could find answers.

I know I will ruffle some feathers by writing about what happened to me in the support groups, the online group and the one provided by Dr. No's office. It is a risk I have decided to take and expect some angry people. I also know there are people who are glad I have spoken up about how some are treated by support groups because they too have been mistreated.

Some people seem so fanatic about the gastric bypass surgery that they want everyone overweight to have one. This is a personal decision and no one should be pressured into it. They should be well informed with all of the pros and cons to the surgery.

It disturbs me to hear that there are Weight Loss Seminars being held to recruit people into having the surgery. There are also advertisements on the television espousing only the benefits of the surgery. This appears to me to be representing a fad diet instead of a personal decision between a patient and their doctor.

The negative reaction I received in the support groups and on-line chat rooms is the reason why I wanted to keep private the names of people who helped me, and graciously allowed me to share their stories in this book, newspaper articles, and in national television interviews. I did not want these fanatics to go after my friends, family, and those that would only talk to me about their experiences if they remained anonymous. I have been told to keep quiet by the "cheerleaders" of this surgery and I won't. Until every person is given the pros as well as the cons of the surgery and is thoroughly informed I will continue to speak up.

I will continue to promote education as the way to inform patients and to keep open the dialogue between all people so we can benefit from each other. There is no reason to attack another person because they are having problems caused by the surgery. If we can learn from each other than we can further help support those who are in need.

9

Family and Friends

Support

I did not tell my friends, or family, about having the gastric bypass surgery before having it done. The only people that knew were my husband and children. My twin sister, Danica, guessed I had the surgery two weeks after I had it since she was throwing up all the time, very nauseous and in pain. Being an identical twin, we have experienced each others illnesses and injuries on several occasions even though we live 1,200 miles apart. She knew it was not about her, but about me, and asked if I had done something to myself.

Like I said before, I am a very private person and not used to revealing personal problems. It just is not my nature and felt it was a matter for only me and my immediate family to know about. Danica knew about my surgery two weeks after I had it and agreed to keep this to herself for several months. I didn't want to burden my sisters and brothers with my problems.

When Dr. No told me he wouldn't reverse the procedure I knew I would need all of their support to help me through the long process in finding help to get my life back.

Danica lived so far away from me yet was there for me when I needed her. She encouraged me to tell all the rest of my brothers and sisters about what I was going through. My father had passed on many years ago and I had very little contact with my mother. When my mother found out about the surgery I had she was very supportive. I always knew I could rely on my family if there were ever a need to do so and now was the time to reach out to them.

I wanted to tell my family and, if need be, ask for their help. I finally believed I wouldn't be burdening them with my problem but rather allowing them to help me. They all know I am a very private person and did not complain about problems so for them to hear what I had been going through surprised most of them.

Some of my family had an idea, but waited until I wanted to talk with them about it and ask for their help. I did not get one negative response, rather their love and support. I knew then that I was not alone on this journey. Three of my siblings were considering having the gastric bypass surgery. After hearing what I was going through, they changed their minds. They felt there was a much better way than to risk their health and life going through this surgery. I am happy to tell you they have found other ways and are now losing weight and are healthy at the same time.

One of my brothers still struggles with his weight and is getting encouragement from the rest of the family to find what will work for him. Until I spoke with him, he had been being pressured by his doctor to have the gastric bypass surgery. He did a great deal of research into this procedure as I did. Listed below are some of the pros and cons we found on the internet, talking with others, and from doctor's offices.

Benefits

Some of the benefits in having the gastric bypass surgery are; weight loss, which may but not always improve conditions including arthritis, sleep apnea, lower back pain, blood sugar levels, and an improved quality of life. There are lists that include more benefits, but this is what I received from Dr. No's office.

Information about the benefits is readily available and often overstated, but the downside of the surgery is not so easy to find. Dr. No told me; only about 1 percent has any serious problems, which I now know is far from the truth. Over half of all the people I have spoken with and the stories I have read from others have had problems due to the bypass operation. (According to Dr Livingston's studies of 800 patients at UCLA, up to 40 percent experienced serious complications)

Most people going into the surgery say they are aware of all the risks and feel they will be one of the lucky ones with no problems. Based on my experience from interviews and letters; the odds are 50 percent or higher you will be in the group that has life threatening ailments. There are those that are happy now with their bypass operation but, how long will that last? Nobody knows for certain. *Many deaths, directly linkable to the gastric bypass are not recorded as related to the gastric bypass surgery as a result of mis-filing them under other categories, such as obesity, organ failure, heart attack and more.*

Negatives

The downside in having the gastric bypass surgery are; risk of heart attack from rapid weight loss and malnutrition, anemia, osteoporosis, risk of auto immune disease like LUPUS and possibly, as some rheumatologists theorize, multiple sclerosis and rheumatoid arthritis, fibromyalgia, nerve damage, ulcers, higher risk of cancer of the throat and stomach, hair loss, severe depression, mal-absorption syndrome, abdominal hernia, hypoglycemia, kidney and liver failure, vomiting, chronic nausea, regaining the weight, lactose intolerance, food allergies, complications from a breakdown in the staple line, stretched stomach outlet, gallbladder disease, damaged metabolism, constipation, diarrhea, increased stress and anxiety disorders, muscle pain, metabolic bone disease, iron deficiencies, weakness, chronic fatigue syndrome, challenged immune system and death. Some of these problems can happen right away, like blood clots which can cause death and others problems and can take years to manifest.

My brother was scared at what he had learned so decided to trust his intuition and not have a WLS, and to find another solution that was less invasive. His doctor is still putting pressure on him to have the gastric bypass surgery, but he feels there has to be another way. Our entire family will help him any way we can. I will not put any pressure on him in any way and neither will other family members. Whatever he decides I will support him one hundred percent and be there for him.

After talking with my family about the gastric bypass surgery and the problems I was having, I decided it was time to talk with my friends. They had been worried for a long time about me yet understood my reluctance to talk about myself. Like my family, they were all very supportive. A few could not understand why I would do something this drastic to myself. I told them I thought I was doing it to improve my health. Instead of feeling great, they saw that I had worse health than before. My friends knew I did not do it to look more attractive; they loved me for who I was and already thought I was beautiful within and on the outside.

When we moved to our present home most of my friends lived quite a long ways away and had not seen me for awhile. Some saw me during the months of losing weight and kept asking me if I had cancer or some other ailment. My face was always pale and I had lost that sparkle in my eyes that was always present before. I met a friend for lunch, or I should say a couple of crackers, and she was shocked when she saw me. Her first words were, "what happened to you, you look so sick and you did not tell me you were ill." I was grateful she did not say, oh, you lost weight. Rather, she asked how my health was. Once I told her what was going on she just hugged me and told me it would be alright. She had never known me to have physical problems or limitations and now that was what was consuming my life.

My family and friends know I am a person with a strong will and will do whatever it takes to get something resolved. The intent of the gastric bypass surgery was to have an improved quality of life, but that turned out to be the furthest from reality. Although I did not make my weight loss goal it was fine by me. It was never a priority to lose weight for vanity. My declining health had made my quality of life worse. Before the surgery, I lived an active normal life, could exercise, run my business, and participate in life. Now it was all I could do to survive each day!

Many people go into this surgery feeling they will not be one of those that "could" have problems or die from it. They feel it is worth it to be thinner and it will improve their self esteem and health. I have to admit that I was one of those people that did not think I would have any problems because of Dr. No's reassurance that the possibility of problems was slim. He said his patients have done very well and saw that I would do just fine. Later, I found this statement to be untrue and I had not been given the full truth about the complications.

I was not willing to give up on improving my health and seeking the truth about the gastric bypass surgery and the reversal. With the support of family and friends I knew I could lean on them at any time. They would also continue to educate themselves about the dangers of this surgery and pass it on to others looking into it. They didn't want me to die or have a life of continuous health problems due to this surgery. I have learned a lot about love, compassion, and support. I know longer have a problem reaching out for help.

Danica

The following is a letter written by my twin sister Danica to show what a family member of someone going through problems with the WLS endures. It is important to have her story in her own words, from her own experience because this surgery doesn't just affect the patient but those they love as well.

Dani is my twin sister and I am so thankful that I am writing about her life instead of her death.

Although I found out about Dani's bypass surgery a couple of weeks following the surgery, my involvement started a few months later when her health had deteriorated. I knew she was unhappy with the way she looked and had gained weight. I also knew that she felt frustrated and didn't know what to do to get the weight off.

Two weeks after she had the gastric bypass surgery she shared with me the ordeal she went through. She was having difficulty keeping food down and was only able to attempt small portions of soft food throughout the day. She started walking after the surgery and was initially gaining some strength.

I was very upset that she had this procedure. If she had talked to me before having the surgery, I would have flown there and talked her out of it!

She had read the research Dr. No had given her on the procedure and felt it was a way of saving her life.

As the months passed I saw my twin sister fading away. My heart was sad and I felt helpless that there wasn't anything I could do. I didn't want to lose her. We made a pact as children not to ever leave each other. Dani's outlook on life was dismal and felt like the Dr. No wasn't listening to her.

I was calling her every day on my breaks at work. I was feeling her slip into a person I didn't recognize. Dani is so strong and able to work through anything. My twin was losing the battle to find out what was wrong.

One day while I was at work, I thought, she needs me and what am I doing here when I could be with her. Dani's husband offered to fly me to their home to take care of her. I talked to the owner of my company and he told me to go. I went to my immediate boss and told her I was booking myself out for two weeks. I left the next day. Dani and her husband met me at the airport. I didn't know my role yet, but I knew I had to be with her.

Dani's whole life became a struggle to live. She would have to remember to take all kinds of pills and tried to keep food down. She became obsessed with food after the surgery, trying all day to get in protein drinks and hoping some of would stay down.

Her beautiful hair was falling out, skin was sagging and her image of herself was still as a very large person. We went clothes shopping to buy her clothes that fit her, yet she was feeling so sick. When we got home, we went into her closet and pull all of her fat clothes and gave them away so that she wouldn't be reminded any more.

She would pull up all her strength to get out of the house and we would go out for a short walk until she was just too weak to go on. Dani would wake up every morning and cry for hours and she felt herself dying. Part of me was dying also.

I knew it was my job to be her advocate. Then I got mad. Enough of Dr. No, who said her problems were in her head. I even went with her to see a therapist, which did nothing, because it wasn't in her head. It was inside of her stomach.

I knew she would need to seek help and we would need her medical records so I encouraged her to call Dr. No's office and ask for a copy, it took several days to get them. The naturopath also wanted a copy of her records to see what exactly was done to her so he could try to give her the supplements to get her health back.

When we received the records and Dani read them over, she saw discrepancies and things she didn't know were done. She felt so bad and cried over the betrayal. I felt helpless too. I felt her despair and my frustration was growing, and I didn't know what to do either. I knew she had to get to another doctor that would evaluate her.

We began to look out of state for a specialist since we had already tried looking for a doctor in the state she lived and no one would help. We soon found out doctors don't like to take on other doctor's patients so the battle began. I looked into specialists where I live and talked to people and kept networking. Dani was even thinking of going to England where someone there was looking into helping her get the procedure reversed.

Dani found a place that is very reputable and qualified in the United States so she wouldn't have to travel far. After finding a doctor that would help we then had to battle with the insurance company. We would move ahead and then hit a setback. Finally when the insurance company realized how ill she was, they gave approval for her to go out of plan.

When I returned home, I continued to call Dani several times a day to check up on her progress. Dani would feel too weak some days to make the calls, but I had her write down the numbers to call and what questions to ask. The word "no" was no longer acceptable.

I gave Dani encouragement to take one day at a time. She would need to move forward in getting the consultation with the new doctor (Dr. Compassion) who would do her reversal, and then, set up an appointment to have testing done before surgery.

I couldn't be with Dani while she went through the testing and the surgery, but my heart would be with her.

This journey has affected me in many ways. I made the decision to get myself healthy and to start taking care of myself. I stand up for myself now and so does she. My twin is back.

The problems people have with the WLS doesn't just affect them, it affects their loved ones as well. My twin sister went through a lot with me and continues to be there for me every day as I will always be there for her.

10

Food Obsession

It had now been eighteen months since having the gastric bypass surgery. Instead of my health problems getting better like Dr. No and his nurse said they would, the problems were getting worse. Besides continued health problems, I had also developed an eating disorder that was consuming my every day life.

I had read about eating disorders, like bulimia and anorexia, but never thought I would have an obsession until now. My life had become consumed with food; can I get it in without vomiting, will I become nauseous if I eat, can I get in protein, fluids, calcium, B-12, vitamins, and will I be in pain if I do eat?

From the moment I got up in the morning until I went to bed at night I thought of little else than "how I was going to get in enough food to live." I continued to try and take in fluids and food very slowly. I was so used to eating cold soup since it took so long between spoonfuls. Without nutrients my health would continue to deteriorate and I worried about this dilemma daily.

Getting in nutrients when I left home to shop for groceries or to get some errands done for my family was a struggle. Sometimes I would take a thermos of pureed soup to drink if I would be out for several hours. Leaving home for any reason took a lot of planning. If I forgot to bring crackers with me or soup in a container, I would have to cut my day short to get home before I ran out of energy. I always had to bring a bowl with me everywhere I went in case I vomited. It became such an ordeal to go outside my home and to have to deal with throwing up in public so I stayed home. It got to the point I left my home only once a week, and then only for an hour at a time.

I wanted to get a job to help pay for some of the medical bills. Unfortunately, who would hire me if I had to frequently run to the bathroom to vomit? An employer wouldn't want me to have a 'bowl' with me all the time either. I had no energy to work even a part-time job let alone working full time like a healthy person would be able to do.

I knew I needed to rest to hold on to any strength I had. Yet, my mind needed something more. I wanted to exercise, it was important to my mental well being. I was not used to a life without activity and for over a year of limited mobility it had taken a toll on me.

I was up to 400 calories a day so I felt I could start some kind of activity. I started taking short walks, one to two miles every other day, but soon had to let that go. I would end up coming home and falling down on the floor several times the rest of the day. My legs would not hold me up and I would end up crying in defeat. I also did not want to be outside on a country road and end up on the ground again, and have to be brought to my car or home. This already happened a few times before and it was embarrassing as well as dangerous. I did not want to become prey for the mountain lion living in the area as I walked along the gravel road.

Walking was also getting more difficult because my bones and muscles throughout my whole body hurt so much. I started taking up to four times the amount of calcium and vitamins, but that did not seem to make a difference with the discomfort. I first noticed my bones and muscles hurting about six months out from my surgery the pain continued to get worse. I had a bone density test before the surgery and I was in great condition, but now, after surgery I was not so sure. I plan on getting regular testing in the future to see if there has been any deterioration.

Since walking any distance was hard on my bones I thought I could try swimming. For years I had been a distance swimmer so thought this would be less stress on my joints and bones, so I went to the recreational center to swim. I started out swimming only four laps the first day, and was having a problem with weakness and dizziness afterwards and asked an attendant if she would help me get some water from my locker. A few days later I went swimming again and increase by laps by four, but afterwards I did not do so good.

My legs gave out in the dressing room and I had to ask an attendant for help. The lady got me some crackers from my locker and after eating a couple I felt strong enough to get ready and go home. I thought maybe I had not had enough food or fluids in before swimming so rested and got some strength back.

A few weeks later I went back to the pool to just swim a couple of laps and relax in the water. I drank some carrot juice before hand to get some fluids and nutrients. I drank carrot juice before and it stayed in so I thought there was not going to be a problem. Within a few minutes of floating in the water I became very nauseous, dizzy, and vomited in the pool. I was so humiliated. The people at the recreational center told me that they could not tell me to not to come back, but advised me to get well before trying to swim again.

I took their advice and will not go back until I know for sure I can use their facilities without risking my health and worry them about liability. Mentally, I was ready to resume some kind of activity, but my body was not physically able to continue with any sort of exercise program. Again, I had to put on hold physical activity and would have to wait until I got stronger.

In the mean time, I continued going to the naturopath. I was already taking several supplements now just to hold on to what little energy I had. The supplements were good for me; the problem was the absorption and the nausea that accompanied just about everything I consumed.

The nausea and vomiting had also prevented me from going out with my husband to dinner or going to friends homes for a meal. Throwing up in public is humiliating if you can't get to the bathroom in time. One time the food came out so fast I threw up in my husband's plate. Needless to say, we left the restaurant right away.

If the restaurant had soup I was alright, as long as it did not have any dairy products in it, otherwise I ate a couple of crackers. I faced the same problem going to friends homes for meals so we turned down any invitations. I did not want to spend time explaining to our friends why I could not eat the meal they prepared. Nor did I want anyone to pity me. I have a lot of pride and was not going to ruin a great evening because I had to lie down from being nauseous or run to their bathroom to vomit.

I could have easily become a prisoner in my home. Too weak to exercise, not enough energy to continue with my business, vomiting and nausea throughout the day and night, muscle and bone pain, hypoglycemia, lactose intolerant, dizziness, heart palpitations, several food allergies, continued hair loss, memory loss, and on top of all that I now needed several crowns replaced on my teeth from all the vomiting and lack of proper nutrition. I was told by Dr. No that I didn't have acids in my stomach to cause my teeth to go bad but he didn't address the lack of nutrients. Lack of absorption of calcium, vitamins, and minerals all play an important roll when it comes to having healthy teeth and gums. I wasn't benefiting from the supplements so it was no surprise I had problems with my teeth and gums as well as bones.

During the first year following the gastric bypass surgery I had also lost one and a quarter inches in height and my cholesterol had still not dropped. My blood pressure and pulse rate continued to be below normal most days. I still took these readings every day with my own cuff. There were times when my blood pressure went up due to stress. The stress from all the problems elevated my blood pressure and I was beginning to think my life would make a good country western song or would top any soap opera story on television.

I wasn't satisfied living my life like a soap opera and it would change, I knew this in my heart. Instead of putting energy into what was not going right with my physical condition, I began putting my energy into what was going right. The small things in life often produce the biggest rewards. A hug from my husband and children, support from friends, and a big kiss from my dogs lifted my spirit. I did not take any of these treasures for granted and cherished the joy in my life, despite any limitations that were present. I greeted the rising sun every morning and thank the Great Spirit and the Goddess Mother Earth for the beauty in all things.

11

My Search

I needed to begin searching for another doctor to help me with my problems after deciding to leave Dr. No and anyone associated with his office. Dr. No was the only one in my area who had any kind of background with the gastric bypass surgery, so I had to look elsewhere to find a qualified doctor to do the reversal. With Danica's help I called several other doctors and they all informed me they did not do the gastric bypass reversal, let alone perform it in the first place. Many doctors I talked with will not even do the gastric bypass because of all the long term follow up care required, and they also felt it was a high risk and unnecessary procedure.

I began running into walls every where I turned. I checked on the internet for doctors with this specialty and sent off e-mails to doctors in St. Louis, Oregon, California, Ohio, Colorado, and Washington State. Most never responded, but the two that did said the gastric bypass was not reversible. I was determined to find help. This was my life at stake and could not just let it go by the wayside.

Over all these months of searching out answers to why my physical health was not getting better I had to keep moving forward. I went to the naturopath and my family physician several times, gynecologist, psychologist every week, checked out support groups, researched the library and internet for anything I could find about the gastric bypass and the reversal. I wrote letters to doctors and asked other people I met with this procedure to get input and advice.

I finally found a doctor in a city near where I live and made an appointment for a consultation. It would be two months before I could see him and that meant another two months of being ill.

I continued with the remedies from the naturopath and hoped they would keep my health from getting any worse than it was.

I was able to leave my house once a week to go grocery shopping and sometimes get in an errand or two, depending on my energy level. Most days were spent in bed or resting in a chair because I had no energy to do any normal daily activities.

One afternoon I was driving past the health food store and felt like there was someone there I needed to connect with. I followed my intuition and went in. At the deli there were a woman and her daughter waiting in line to get their food. We began small talk about the different salads and I told her I could only get in soup at this time. I revealed to her my situation and was looking for a qualified doctor who could help me. Up to this point I had not told anyone except my family and friends about the surgery, so this was new territory for me. Like I said before, I was not ashamed of having the gastric bypass surgery, just not accustomed to revealing personal matters regarding my life.

There are no coincidences, the woman and her daughter at the deli were there for a reason, and so was I. The woman looked at me and asked if I was a student of metaphysics and I said, yes. The reason why she asked me this question is because, if I was metaphysical, I would understand what she was about to tell me and not dismiss it as being weird to get an intuitive reading. She proceeded to tell me she felt there was a doctor who could help me, the first initial of his last name, and which state he was in, but I would have to do some searching to find him.

That afternoon, I went on the internet and looked in the state she said I would find the doctor. Now, I am considered computer challenged so it took awhile, but I finally found Dr. Compassion and his phone number. This was a very prestigious institution and I was nervous as to whether he would even be taking any new patients, but I got up my nerve and made the call. I spoke with a most wonderful nurse who told me I could get a consultation with him and gave me his qualifications. His background was exactly what I was looking for so I made the appointment. My husband booked our flight that afternoon.

I decided to use this time to continue researching the pros and cons of the gastric bypass reversal. I spent days looking in the library, bookstores, and on line to find anything about the reversal and came up with a little information. There was one article on the internet and that is all I found after many days of searching. With the expertise of this new doctor, I was going to wait and see what he had to say.

12

Insurance Approval

While I waited for the day to come for my consultation visit, I called my insurance company to see about medical coverage. Dr. Compassion was out of network and I needed approval to go to him. After hearing about my situation and lack of experts in my area the insurance company gave the approval.

The woman I spoke with at the insurance company was most interested in my case and asked if I would be willing to share what I had gone through. I thought this kind of odd, but I went ahead and answered her questions.

She later revealed to me why all the questions and then I understood. *She has a friend who is dying from the gastric bypass and she did not know how to comfort her.* Her friends' physician told her he could not do the gastric bypass reversal at the present time.

The woman's body had been in starvation for so long that she no longer had the strength to make it through the surgery and all her organs were failing. If they could build up her body she would be able to withstand the long surgery. She had stomach tubes to feed her and now they were waiting to see if she would make it.

The woman's physical problems did not happen overnight. She thought she would get better in time and her blood work up showed everything was going fine, even though all the tests showed she was at the bottom of the normal range. It took time before her blood tests caught up to what was really going on in her body. My heart went out to this woman and I hope she made it, but the prognosis was not good.

The woman from the insurance company understood what I was going through and planned to continue to support her friend, even if it was just to hold her hand and give her love. She was also willing to share information with me that they get in from doctor's offices regarding the gastric bypass surgery.

The main physical problem some insurance companies are seeing is heart failure due to rapid weight loss, and a high incidence of kidney and liver problems. The list of problems went on and on and it was enough to make me wonder why all this information is not made available to the public.

The woman at the insurance company said, "Doctor's are putting through these problems as related to morbid obesity rather than complications for the gastric bypass surgery." Some doctor's offices appear to be not showing their current and potential patients accurate data. I can't help wonder if it is all about the money or if many of these doctors do not have the statistics from other physicians. Ignorance in this case should not be acceptable. Doctors performing any kind of surgery should have all the information available or else they shouldn't be doing the surgery, regardless if it is the gastric bypass or any other surgery.

The woman at the insurance company gave me a lot of information and was compassionate as well. Most of us looking for information about the gastric bypass hear wonderful success stories and those on television espousing how happy they are with their surgery. There had to be more people out there that are having problems, and I wanted to learn more while I waited for my consultation visit with Dr. Compassion.

13

Dr. Compassion

Consultation

My husband and I arrived at Dr. Compassion's office for the consultation regarding the gastric bypass reversal. It was a long day of traveling and we were tired. Yet, we were anxious to get answers to our questions.

I brought with me a copy of all my medical records as well as a list of questions and gave them to Dr. Compassion. We sat in his office and went over everything I had given him. At one point during the consultation I began to cry and Dr. Compassion reached out and put his hand on mine. He said he would help me anyway he could and was there for me. After meeting this new doctor and speaking with him I decided I would call him, Dr. Compassion.

Dr. Compassion did not patronize me or treat me with disrespect as I had been treated by others. He treated me with the respect I deserved. He reviewed all my records, answered my questions, and then gave me two options. One was to go right to the gastric bypass reversal, and the other was to go through an entire work up, which included tests, and to be seen by his support team. It was up to me to choose which plan of action I wanted to pursue. I wanted to try and avoid surgery if there was a problem that could be fixed without another intrusive procedure so I choose the entire work up option.

We returned home and waited to hear from Dr. Compassions' office regarding a schedule for me to return for the tests. *I finally had hope and a plan of action!* I had made up my mind to go with Dr. Compassion so I cancelled my consultation appointment with the doctor located in a nearby city.

Within a couple of weeks I received my schedule in the mail and made plans to return for the tests and to meet with Dr. Compassions' support team. The wait was not easy, questions and concerns kept running through my mind. Would anything be found that could be easily taken care of without surgery or would surgery be the only way for me to get my health back? All I could do now is try to take care of myself and get lots of rest.

Resting is not an easy thing for me to do and like all mothers there is plenty to do with a family. Just standing up was a problem because of the dizziness. I often would have to sit right back down or risk falling. Bumping into walls from the dizziness was also a problem.

By this point it had been over a year since having the gastric bypass surgery. I felt like I had been a burden to my family but they did not see it that way. Still, it bothered me to have them watch me go through all these problems. I had always taken care of everyone else and now it was my turn to ask for help which I did without guilt. I did what I could do and had to let the rest go, or wait until someone else picked up the work I normally did. For someone that likes everything clean and in order this was not an easy task to relinquish to someone else but there was no other choice. It was a good lesson for me and watching my husband and sons do all the cleaning was rather nice.

14

Dr. Compassion

Medical Testing

With airline tickets in hand, hotel reservations complete, and bags packed I was ready for several days of testing and evaluations by Dr. Compassion and his team of experts. I was told by the airlines security at the airport was tight and they would be checking my bags. I was surprised to have been asked about the contents of my carry on bag after it went through their scanner. There were several bottles of medications, tinctures from my naturopath, vitamins, calcium, and a variety of supplements. I assured them that I was not a drug dealer or a pharmacist and needed all of this for my health. I had my medical records with me and schedule from Dr. Compassion's office so they passed me through without further questions. The woman who did the scanning of my bags just looked at me and said, "I hope you get better and will not have to take all this stuff for the rest of your life." I just smiled and moved on.

Along with all the medications and supplements in my carry on bag, I also had to take with me crackers and cold soup to eat during the flight. Airports and airlines do not have any food I could eat, especially pureed soup. I was able to pass through their scanner with plastic containers on this trip. Traveling was a real chore but at least I was able to drink something.

My husband could not take time off from work for this evaluation trip, so one of my sisters, Joan, came with me on this trip. Joan writes about her experience with me in an article she wrote that is included later on.

Joan was coming from another state so we timed our flights to meet at the airport in Arizona where Dr. Compassion's office was.

From the day I first told Joan about having the gastric bypass surgery and what I had been going through, she was absolutely supportive, as well as the rest of my family, in my quest to get help. Joan did not want me to be by myself during these days of testing and it was a relief for my husband to know I would not be alone.

Joan and I arrived at Dr. Compassion's office to begin my testing. My first appointment was with the dietician. She reviewed the medications and supplements I was taking along with the foods I was eating. Many suggestions were made to help me get in more nutrients. I was to puree the food, including all soups that had vegetables, for one month and continue with all my supplements. I had already been doing this but would continue to follow this suggestion.

My next appointment was at the gastrointestinal department for an upper endoscope procedure. I had been fasting since the day before and not very steady on my feet. This is where Joan was able to help me from falling over from weakness. I was given medication and the procedure was done with no discomfort at all. Joan drove me back to our hotel for soup and rest before the next day of testing.

On day two of testing, my first appointment was with the endocrinology therapist. We talked for over an hour about everything I had gone through since having the gastric bypass surgery. It wasn't easy to hold back the tears during this session because I had to re-live many experiences that were difficult to go through. She wrote up her evaluation and gave it to Dr. Compassion.

Later that afternoon, I went back to the endocrinology department to meet with a physician's assistant for history taking and a physical exam. After this was done another doctor came in with two assistants to review the history that I had given to the assistant and her findings from the exam.

Blood was found in my stool so I would need a colonoscopy test. There wasn't time, so I would make that appointment with a local physician once I returned home. When the interview with the doctor and his associates was over a report was written and given to Dr. Compassion.

On the third and last day of testing, I went to the Radiology Department for a test to evaluate my colon and small intestines. They told me it would take about at least an hour and up to four hours for this test. I drank the barium and waited for twenty to thirty minutes and went back for the x-rays. The barium had already gone through my system. They told me it went through rapidly and that I was free to go.

Later, when I got home I received a report from the endocrinologist that stated the person performing the test found a small hernia inside that was not picked up at the time I had the barium procedure. It was unfortunate I was released too early or further testing would have been done.

That afternoon I went to see Dr. Compassion to review all the tests done over the last three days. He went over everything and the tests showed nothing conclusive as to why I frequently vomited, up to eight times a day, and had chronic nausea. There was something wrong, but what it was nobody knew. Dr. Compassion was not giving up on me and told me he would consult with other experts to see if they could shed some light as to what might be going on with my body. *The team all agreed that I was not informed enough about the gastric bypass prior to my surgery.* I totally agreed with that finding, but there was nothing I could do about it now. I decided I would go home and wait until Dr. Compassion consulted with other doctor's about my situation.

Joan and I left for the airport to return to our homes. It had been a long three days and I was tired and discouraged. I wanted something minor found that was obvious and could be easily remedied.

Dr. Compassion and all his team were great and treated me with respect. I could not have asked for a better team to work with. I was thankful that I now had a team that was not going to give up on me.

On the plane going home I could not hold in my emotions from the last three days any longer. I was so tired and had little to eat during the flight, I began to cry. I was worn out. I have never cried in public and have always been able to put on a happy face, but not this time. It was night time and dark in the plane, so I just let it out, quietly. The flight attendants were so nice to me and offered me something to drink and eat. I tried to eat a few crackers, but vomited them up. One flight attendant in particular was so caring and asked me if she could do anything for me. She thought I might be upset about the security on the plane because of the tragic events that occurred on September 11th, 2001 in NYC. I assured her that was not the case and I was just tired from the trip and wanted to get home to my family.

Once I got home and back to my serene surroundings, I was able to get in some pureed food and fluids. I spent several days relaxing to get my strength back and to wait for Dr. Compassion to get back to me with any information he could fine to assist me.

In the mean time, I did have the colonoscopy test when I got home and results were benign. The colonoscopy specialist told me he had always been against any WLS, but was beginning to change his mind after reading about patients being happy with the procedure. He does not do any WLS and had patients who have had problems, but had not seen anything like what I had been going through. The colonoscopy specialist sat and talked with me about what I had gone through after having the WLS. After listening to my story he said, "*I will never recommend this surgery to any of my patients*". He stated, "*As a doctor, I had a hard time finding any information about the downside to the surgery and could imagine how hard it is for potential patients to find it.*"

A lack of information available to doctors and patients is one of the biggest problems facing people seeking the WLS. This should not be happening. But, it is! When more people with WLS problems get their story out to the public, then those who are looking into having the surgery can make an informed decision.

15

Vision Quest

While I waited for Dr. Compassion to inform me of any findings that could help me resolve the problems, I decided it was time to go on a Vision Quest.

I am part Native American, Seneca Tribe, and follow the traditions of my heritage. While in meditation, I heard from the spirits of the Grandmothers; they are the wise elders who are there for all Mother Earths children. I learned that the answers I seek are within and I would find them in solitude. When my spirit calls for me to do something to further my growth, I listen. Going within is the way I find peace and to learn more about myself.

I spent hours sitting in my Medicine Wheel, the place we experience all aspects of life and heal by learning about ourselves. Every spoke on the Wheel is an aspect of the self and the center is the core of our spirit.

I also have a Sweat Lodge that represents the womb of Mother Earth and to go into the Lodge is to heal the mind, body, and spirit. The Lodge is a dome structure made out of willow and covered with blankets. After crawling inside the lodge the hot lava rocks are brought in and the door is shut. In complete darkness the sweat begins and prayers of healing are shared. It is a place where I am nurtured and able to release what no longer is needed in my life. I have very briefly described what goes on in a Sweat Lodge and it is important for me to mention this because it was an integral part of my healing process.

Each one of us finds a way that gives us comfort and is to be honored and respected. I believe we are all here on Mother Earth to embrace each other, differences and all. To give aid to others when needed and to receive help when offered is something we all can strive to achieve.

After going to the Medicine Wheel and Sweat Lodge I was ready to head off into the mountains to find a spot where I could be completely alone to find my answers. I stayed outside in the elements for days until I learned what I needed to know.

A Vision Quest is a very private experience so I will not go into the details of my journey. I will say, I learned about myself and what I needed to do to get back into balance with all aspects of the self. Taking time to contemplate the purpose of ones life is an ongoing process that allows personal growth.

A spiritual path is important, no matter what path you choose, to help give strength during every day life. Like every sister and brother of Mother Earth we all have a purpose and gifts to give others that will help them as well as ourselves. The Goddess Mother Earth gives me this strength to preserver through the most trying times and the best of times.

All experiences make up who I am and I have no regrets. I have not denied myself the emotions that have come up during all these months and learning how I deal with them is up to me. There is always a lesson to learn from all situations and I have chosen to live a positive life, and not dwell on any anger or negativity. If I let Dr. No take control over my emotions, then he wins. And, I won't let that happen.

The decision to have the gastric bypass surgery was not a mistake, despite all the problems I have endured. It gave me the ability to learn a very big lesson. It is always a personal choice whether to live in the past or to move forward. I can't change the past. But I can make the most of what I have learned. It's obvious I didn't give up my trust about doctors since I was putting my life and trust in Dr. Compassion. I was deserving of the best care possible and never gave up hope that I would get better once I found a solution to my problem. The knowledge I have gained through this lesson can now be shared with others, it is time.

16

The Reversal Decision

Dr. Compassion and I spoke about his consultations with other doctor's regarding the problems I was having with the RNY. They concluded that I had a narrowed gastrojejunostomy (i.e. the opening between my stomach and small gut had narrowed probably due to adhesions) as well as a probable foreign body around the gastrojejunostomy (probably a silastic ring commonly done in this variation of the gastric bypass) from the Fobi pouch procedure. It was decided that I would undergo the takedown of my gastric bypass. I was counseled regarding the possibilities of regaining weight. We also discussed the possibility of re-doing of my gastric bypass. However, I wanted my anatomy returned to normal as much as was possible. Once Dr. Compassion performed the reversal he would know for certain the cause of my poor health.

Dr. Compassion knew how much I wanted my health to improve. Nothing I tried was working and it was time to take the most drastic option. I could not live with malnutrition the rest of my life and *felt my life wouldn't last another year if I did not do something to change this situation.*

The decision to have the reversal was not made in haste. From the time I first started exploring the option of having my gastric bypass reversed to this point in time it had been eight months. During this eighteen month period I had done everything asked of me, and more, to improve my health. I could have just done nothing and put up with a declining health. Instead, I took a very active role to take back control of my life.

At eighteen months, my muscles and bones hurt more than ever. I had a choice to sit in my chair and wait to die, or find out what was going on. Dr. Caring took blood tests and they showed I was still in normal range, but at the bottom, and continuing to drop from previous tests.

Despite the nausea I was trying to add in more food. But, I wasn't getting better. I had to wait for approval from the insurance company to get the reversal. I was concerned that if I didn't have the reversal soon, I wouldn't have the strength to endure the surgery. I felt time was running out for me.

Dr. Compassion put through the required medical necessity letter to my insurance company for the reversal. He was reluctant at first to put through the medical necessity but after talking with me he decided to put it through. In a few weeks I received confirmation that I had been approved for surgery.

When I got the news I had so many emotions running through me. I was apprehensive about going through another surgery, but if it enabled me to have my life back I was willing to take the risk. There really wasn't much of a choice, I wanted to live.

Getting the good news of the approval for the reversal left me with such elation that I called my family right away and they were one hundred percent behind me. I had hope once again for a healthy life and was excited to have the surgery to reverse the gastric bypass so I could move forward.

Dr. Compassion's surgery schedule had already been booked for the next two months and I was on a waiting list. After two months went by I received my schedule for the gastric bypass reversal. It finally was going to happen and I had felt such a relief to be able to make plans for my future. It had taken one month to get the consultation, another month to get the testing, and then a six month wait to get the reversal.

All the plans to go to this other city for the reversal were made the day I got my schedule from Dr. Compassion and his team. My sister, Joan, and a friend were going to be there for me, as well as a great team of specialists. This friend, I will call her Joy, is trained in the Hawaiian Healing Ways called Loma-Loma and said she would be happy to fly there to work with me. One conversation with Joy and you would see why I give her this name. Joy brings love and light to each person she comes in contact with. Her laughter gives comfort to my spirit, and her wisdom and ability to heal will help my body.

I had the best doctor I could find, and the support of family, friends, and my therapist to be there for me.

I was going into this with a team that supported me in every way. There would also be those with me in spirit since they could not be there physically. I knew I would feel their spirit and healing energy with me throughout my journey. I felt blessed.

17

Gastric Bypass

Reversal

Doctors usually refer to a reversal as a 'takedown' of the gastric bypass procedure. A true reversal puts you back exactly the way you were before having the WLS. A 'takedown' will put the patient back as close as possible to the way they were before the WLS.

In my case, Dr. Compassion called it a 'takedown' since he could not reconnect the pouch to the same place where it was cut from the original stomach. In Dr. Compassion's judgment the pouch would be reconnected to the side of my stomach and possible removal of some of the intestines.

I refer to my gastric bypass 'takedown' as a reversal since it is a word better understood my most readers not familiar with all the terms used with WLS.

It also made sense to me to use the word 'reversal' since I did get back the functions I had before the gastric bypass surgery. I would not be put back exactly the way I was before and I do have permanent damage, but it is close and I do have the ability to absorb nutrients again.

I decided to go into detail about the gastric bypass reversal because it is important to know before having the gastric bypass surgery that complications can arise and what you might have to go through to get your health back. I didn't want to just say I had the surgery and it was over, but to give an account of what I went through because it was part of my journey to regaining my health.

No two people will experience surgery and recovery the exact same way. My story is one example and there are others that I have spoken with that went through similar experiences with their reversal. Not one of them has expressed any regret about having their gastric bypass or any other WLS reversed.

One thing we all had in common was being told *we would gain all our lost weight back and we would be unhappy.* Those of us that have had the reversal are happy we made that choice. Many have said, "I have my life back and will try another, more healthy way, of losing weight and keeping it off". Some do gain back some weight, others gain back all of it, some even loose more weight, and then there are others that maintain their weight loss. No two patients are the same. To those that need the reversal it doesn't matter about the weight because they will lose their life if they didn't have the procedure.

One of the reasons why there is weight gain is that the metabolism has been slowed down due to the months or years of eating very small amounts of food. Weight gain can also have to do with genetics.

Those I have been in contract with still would have the reversal despite some weight gain. Additionally, I have seen many who had a WLS and no reversal, yet they gained all their weight back, and more.

I was counseled about the possibility of weight gain after the reversal and was more concerned with my health so I decided to move ahead with the surgery.

My sister Joan picked me up at the airport two days before my gastric bypass reversal surgery. I would have a day of rest and a day of testing before the surgery. I came from and area of snow and Joan came from an area of rain, so the warm weather was a welcome relief. We also had time to spend by the pool and soak up some sun before I would have to spend several days indoors.

My husband had a medical situation at home to tend to and was unable to come with me on this trip. It was very hard on both of us since we had never been apart for two weeks in over 30 years. However, he was able to call me every day. I wouldn't be alone since Joan and Joy would be with me to give their loving support and healing energy.

Joan brought me to the hospital for testing the next day and all went smoothly. Before checking into the hospital the following morning I had to choke down an awful tasting liquid laxative drink.

Besides drinking the laxative the night before the surgery and again the next morning, many thoughts about the surgery were going through my head. Dr. Compassion had gone over the days testing with me and talked with me about my decision to have the reversal.

From what I had heard from others who had the reversal I expected Dr. Compassion to question my decision and even try to talk me out of it. He did ask me if I was sure I wanted the takedown and I knew in my head and my heart that it was the right decision for me, yet I was still a bit nervous because it was major surgery. I don't know anyone who hasn't been nervous before going into surgery, but I also felt relieved that the struggle to get through one day at a time would soon be over.

To get rid of some of the nervous energy I was feeling about the surgery, I spent time meditating before going to sleep. Meditating helps calm the mind, body, and spirit and that will bring clarity to any matter set before you to resolve. I truly believed I would not be able to live more than a year if I kept on the way I was going. It was an inner knowing and I trusted my intuition about this decision for the reversal and everything inside of me said to go forward with the procedure. I had spent many months preparing myself for the reversal so I was ready to get on with my life.

At 6:00 a.m. the following morning I checked into the hospital. Joan and Joy stayed with me as the nurses prepared me for surgery. I had an epidural put into my back, IV started, and vital signs taken.

Before going into surgery the nurse informed me I could not wear my medicine bag in with me. I have always been able to wear it in with me during other surgeries in my life and did not want to take it off this time, but they were adamant that I was not allowed to wear it. My medicine bag carries my spiritual medicine and is to be kept with me at all times. In my heart I knew my spirit would be strong and I would be protected so I held it to my heart and then gave it to Joan to hold for me. She is someone I trusted completely to hold it in safekeeping until it could be returned to me.

After giving my medicine bag to Joan for safekeeping I was taken to the operating room and don't remember anything until I woke from the surgery. It was a seven hour operation and all went well. A nurse kept Joan and Joy updated every couple of hours. Joan had kept my husband and family updated by phone as to how the surgery was progressing.

Dr. Compassion described to Joan my surgery as a "humpty dumpty" surgery since he had to lay all my intestines out on a table and then put me back together again.

After the surgery was over Dr. Compassion explained to Joan and Joy what had taken place during the procedure. There was a problem found and all my problems weren't in my head but resulted from the RNY gastric bypass surgery. The tests before my surgery showed a narrowing of the opening where the ring had been put on, but it became clear during the surgery as to why I was vomiting all the time. *The silastic ring had been put on too tight and it also rolled inwards, pinching the stoma, whenever anything other than liquids was swallowed.* This was the reason why

I would throw up so often if I tried to eat food, even though I chewed it to the consistency of applesauce. There still was no answer as to why I had chronic nausea. But, at least now I found out there WAS a problem that was remedied with the reversal.

A small part of my intestines also had to be removed because of blockages and adhesions that never showed up on any of the tests, including an endoscope procedure.

Dr. No kept telling me it was in my head, but now I knew for sure there was a physical problem that would never have gotten better with time. If I had kept on the way I was, I would never have been able to consume anything other than liquids which weren't giving me the nutrients to sustain my life. I couldn't even tolerate pureed foods, so I was left with clear liquids before the reversal. It was best for me to have the gastric bypass reversed and not to just have the ring taken off. I needed to be able to absorb nutrients again and this was accomplished by reconnecting the bottom part of my stomach. It was unhealthy for me to stay in malnutrition any longer.

In some cases I have read about, the removal of the ring is sufficient to alleviate the problems, but every situation is not the same and this decision is up to the patient and their doctor. I had discussed this option with Dr. Compassion before having the reversal and decided it was best to go with reversing the procedure. I knew when I woke up in recovery my body had been repaired and I would not have to go through anymore vomiting and nausea.

From the moment I awoke from the gastric bypass reversal surgery I knew it was the right decision for me. When Joan told me the doctor found the problem I was so happy to finally have an answer. I knew there was something wrong all along but couldn't get anyone to believe me. Every day that passed in the hospital I gained strength. The healing process was moving forward and I felt so much better to get my life back. An important part of my recovery included family and friends who were there for me every step of the way.

I was told in the recovery room I would be going to the intensive care unit for a day before going to my room. At that time, Joan made sure I had my medicine bag back. It meant the world to me to have part of who I am back with me.

All I remember of being in intensive care was the itching I had all over. The nurse gave me Benadryl® for the allergic reaction I was having to the preservative in the epidural. The itching stopped, but the Benadryl® left me completely zoned. I was grateful that Joan and Joy were there with me to make sure I was getting the best care possible.

By the second day after surgery, I was in my room, and just laid there and didn't get up since the medication had me pretty wiped out.

On the third day after surgery, I was brought to radiology and drank some foul tasting liquid, and then had an x-ray taken to make sure there weren't any leaks. Leaking of the stomach acid can spread toxins throughout the body. The x-ray showed no leaking and I was happy to get that good news.

Later that day, after the x-ray procedure, I was experiencing a lot of pain, so the nurse checked my epidural to see if something was wrong. She couldn't see for sure if it came out, so a pain specialist arrived to check it and sure enough it was out. Instead of putting it back in they hooked me up to a morphine pump and I was soon out of pain.

When the tape around the epidural was taken off it took a strip of skin with it. I have sensitivity to tape so it didn't feel good having it taken off and it left my back with a line of blisters. The sheets on a hospital bed are not the most comfortable so Joan brought in the softest sheets and put them on my bed which helped tremendously. My back didn't rub against stiff sheets so the blisters from the removal of the tape healed very fast.

Once I had the morphine pump working, I was out of pain, which was mainly from gas. I got up the nerve to look at my incision. I had expected to see staples holding me together. Instead there was this smooth line running down my stomach. Dr. Compassion had taken the time and his expertise and used dissolvable stitches.

He had also inserted a gastric tube in my left side. It was put in as a precautionary measure to feed me in the event I needed to be fed. I never had to be fed through the tube but since my history of chronic vomiting it was insert. For the entire stay in the hospital the gastric tube drained fluid from my stomach into a bag. When I left the hospital the tube was detached from the bag and capped. I would then carefully clean around it and keep it dry for six weeks, at which time I would have it removed.

During the next couple of days, Joan and Joy stayed with me and helped in so many ways. It is hard to put into words how much they meant to me by being there. Before Joy had to continue on with her journey of offering her energy healing work to others, she and Joan did a session on me. Together they brought in universal energy to help heal my body and it helped me bring balance to my mind, body and spirit.

The amount of morphine I needed had decreased and I even was able to wash my hair in the sink and have sponge baths with Joan's help. I also felt the many prayers of healing sent to me by my family and friends. I talked with my husband every day and felt like he was there next to me throughout the entire stay in the hospital.

My sister Shara flew in to celebrate her birthday with me and Joan. I hadn't seen her in twelve years so her visit lifted my spirits. Shara wasn't seeing me look my best, but that didn't matter. She was there for me and supported me through this journey. We won't let distance separate us again and we see how important it is to be there for each other during the best of times and through those times when we choose to experience challenges that allow us to grow. Life is full of obstacles, some small and some big, but the process working through any of them is the same. Take one step at a time and keep moving forward, that is how I lead my life every day.

The step I had before me at this time was to pass gas, and I was determined to do my part in making that happen by walking as much as I could, without overdoing it. I was feeling better and doing a great deal of walking, but had to stay in the hospital until my bowels started working. One nurse thought she heard a little rumbling one day and the next day it was very quiet, so I had to wait for that great day when I would pass gas.

Day after day, I would walk and walk trying to get the gas to move through my system; nevertheless I still had a smile on my face. One nurse asked me why I was smiling, and I replied, "I am just so happy to be put back the way I was meant to be, and felt so much better that I didn't have much to be sad about". I hadn't realized until I had the reversal how bad I really had felt until the symptoms were all gone. There wasn't any nausea or vomiting.

The only time I wasn't very happy was when I had to have my IV changed. My veins aren't the greatest so finding one has always been difficult for the nurses. Once they had tried three times to get an IV in, so a specialist was brought in and she was able to find the only vein left in my arms. My arms were bruised. This IV would be my last hope before they would have to take more drastic measures to get fluids and medication in. Luckily, it lasted the two days that were needed.

I finally passed gas on the eighth day after surgery. It is normal to take between eight to ten days after having the reversal to get the bowels working again so I was right on target.

During those eight days I didn't have water or food so I was looking forward to getting in some fluids. I was allowed to put water on my lips and brush my teeth several times a day. Having clean teeth, washed hair, sponge bath, clean gown, and a foot massage adds some normalcy to being in a hospital. I also brought a c.d. player and put on soothing music.

I was going to bring along some Reggae music, but thought I would want to get up and dance before I was ready for such activities. So I saved that music for later.

When I finally passed gas, I did feel like dancing, I was so happy. I was given clear liquids that night and the next day.

Before leaving the hospital on the morning of the tenth day, I was able to say goodbye to some of the nurses that took care of me. As with any hospital, some nurses are more compassionate than others. Most of the ones I had were great and understood why I made the decision to have the reversal. One nurse told me she had worked at a hospital in the Midwest where they reversed all of the weight loss surgeries.

Dr. Compassion and some of his associates came by twice a day to check up on me, and I always had a nurse or one of the patient care assistants there when I needed anything. The nurses took care of my medical needs and Joan took care of all the rest. I especially liked having an extra warmed blanket put on me before trying to going to sleep. I didn't sleep much at night, so I would take walks in the hallways when all was quiet.

The nurses didn't have to encourage me to get up and walk since I don't like being in a bed for any length of time. I was able to push the pole carrying the gastric bag and morphine machine and go outside as often as I wanted. Every day, I would take walks to the gift shop to check out clothes. Shopping is fun no matter what condition you're in, and it gave me an excuse to get out of my room.

One time, I thought how tempting it would be to stand on the sidewalk and hold my thumb out to get a ride out of there. It wasn't that I didn't like it there; it is just a matter of staying indoors when I enjoy the outdoors so very much. I gained strength from breathing fresh air and watching the little birds eating small seeds from the ground around me. Mother Earth is rejuvenating and healing so getting outside was just what I needed.

On the last day, I was given some scrambled eggs before checking out. I was able to keep the eggs down without feeling nauseous or throwing up. This was the first time in eighteen months that I didn't have those feelings and my eyes filled with tears of joy!

Joan helped me dress and pack up all my personal belongings. I was given instructions about medications and how to clean around my gastric tube which I would have for the next six weeks. It was time to leave the hospital, the day I had been looking forward to.

After Joan and I left the hospital, we went shopping for food I could have while we stayed another two days at the hotel. Dr. Compassion wanted me to stay in the area an extra two days before getting on the plane to go home as a precaution. In case anything went wrong I would be close to the hospital, and it also gave me time to get rest at the hotel before traveling home.

The hotel we stayed at had a kitchen, making it much easier to prepare the pureed food I could have. The steak and shrimp Joan had for dinner looked and smelled so good, but I was just happy to have any kind of food without being sick.

The food I was now able to get in gave my body the nutrients it was craving. I had more energy and strength than I have had for the last eighteen months. I knew I was getting weaker day by day before the reversal, but hadn't realized how much better I would feel immediately after surgery. I had expected it to take several weeks to get stronger, but once I had gotten in food that my body could absorb the results surprised me. My body was responding quickly which allowed me to be active.

Walking wasn't a struggle and I didn't fall down from weakness. I was also able to take walks outside to the pool where I could soak my feet and get some sun on my face. It was good to be free from the IV's, and the taking of my blood pressure and temperature every couple of hours. My life was coming together in a balanced and harmonious way.

After two days of getting rest at the hotel, Joan and I were ready to go leave for our homes. Joan drove me to the airport and arranged for wheelchair assistance to get me to the ticket counter and boarding area. It would be a long day of traveling and I didn't want to get too tired so asking for help at the airport wasn't a problem.

Joan and I parted at the security area. I felt sad seeing her leave, she had been a great deal of help and a wonderful sister companion. I will always be grateful for all the help Joan gave me. She made my hospital room cheerful by bringing in flowers, soft bedding, and a beautiful wall hanging, making sure all my needs were being taken care of. Joan and the rest of my family and friends continue to support me as my journey to a healthy life moves forward.

The following is a story written by Joan. I will leave it in her own words as I did with the story written by Danica. It is important for the reader to understand how this surgery impacts the patient's family and friends. Therefore, I have included Joan's story in her own words.

Joan

Joan is another one of my sisters that played an important role in my search for help and recovery besides Danica. She went with me for testing before I had the takedown and was also with me during my hospital stay. The following story is in her words:

> Joanie, yes, this is Dani, hi how are you, you don't sound very well is something wrong? She bursts into tears as she could barley speak as she said "Joanie I didn't tell you the truth about what kind of surgery I had". I said I knew that, as the family had already came to their own conclusion as to why our very private, spiritually centered sister seemed to be showing signs of mental instability and extreme weakness in her physical body.

> She had not eaten in days and if she had eaten she would almost immediately throw up the tablespoon of food that she worked an hour trying to swallow. Dani, you must get to the doctor or at least call him and I am going to call you back to see what he said. The doctor came back with a despairing response, "if you can hold a little water down then you're O.K. and the hospital would only send you back home if you came in". Dani

could barley walk; cried for hours and showed signs of deep despair but according to the doctor she was O.K.

My body was vibrating with contempt for this doctor who had his own agenda and showed such disregard for my sister. Having had two husbands that had died as a result of doctors not listening to their patients I was familiar with the feelings that were inundating me and I was scared to death for her at this point.

Over the next few days the family stayed in very close contact with each other as spoke to her husband to plan a path of recovery for Dani. Her twin flew to Dani's home to help anyway possible and to see how bad she really was. The family did wonder if she was just losing it and needed a psychologist. Yes, she needs a psychologist, a doctor, a surgeon and anyone else that would help her.

With her families support she sought out a doctor of naturopath as well as a therapist, and though there were signs of relief we new we were not getting to the core of the problem. Although Dani is one of the most determined people she was not going to will herself back to health. The family discussed the options and we knew that we needed to get her to the best doctor that western medicine offered, no matter what it cost. Her husband and boys were supportive of her, as they desperately wanted their mother and wife back so they could enjoy life together again.

Dani found it inside herself one more time to seek the help that she knew she needed. It took a month before getting a consultation, another month before testing, and then another six months before having the reversal. Our phones rang constantly to show support, love and sheer determination that we would not stop until she had her life back again.

We meet at the airport and off we went to the clinic for the first batch of testing. The next three days were filled with various appointments and procedures. She was weak and vomiting on a regular basis so we waited at the hotel for the test result to come back.

Having had some medical training and my life's experiences as a point of reference I could pretty well asses what the doctors were implying. They inferred that she was o.k. and she should eat slower and work with a psychologist. As the doctor told her nothing was physically wrong with her you could feel her despair. I held my tongue and dropped down to my soul and asked Spirit for wisdom. I knew she wasn't crazy as I had been with her for several days and I knew she was already doing everything they had just recommended. I wanted to scream, are you not listening to her, she is sick. Yes, she has mental issues, she is starving to death and the nutrients that the naturopath has her on were keeping her levels up enough to keep her out on complete malnutrition and a total breakdown.

THANK GOD the doctor trusted his intuition and left room for the possibility that it wasn't all mental and wanted to keep in touch with her, we left with what appeared to be little hope.

Although the sisters in our family have chosen different paths of enlightenment we were united in One Spirit over the next few months. We spoke that we often felt that we were holding her spirit for her until her body could support it again. I felt that she put herself in a place that she could trust her sister's love for her. She gave me a beautiful piece of green amber while we were together and I have worn it everyday since to visualize the healing that we wanted to take place. Her radical procedure awoke all kinds of suppressed emotions in our family. I know that I had briefly thought of having the operation and several others and expressed the same thoughts. We had no judgment of Dani, as we understood her reasons for choosing the procedure. Six out of seven siblings are obese and have been most of our lives. Several family members have had success by opting to do it the old fashion way since Dani's experience and eat less while working out more.

As the long days progressed into months we saw no improvement as the doctors took a closer look and presented a diagnosis for her condition that prove to be accurate.

One can't even embrace the emotions that the entire family felt when we heard the news that the reversal was approved and the procedure would be preformed. Plans were made and plans were changed as we dealt with Dani and my family needs. The men stayed at home while Dani, I, and a dear woman that I love as a mother headed off to be together. All of us came from different states and when we met we embraced, as we all knew within ourselves what our purpose was. I prepared for a ten to fourteen day stay as well as surgery for my sister.

Joy and I waited for seven plus hours with updates about Dani's progress. Not a lot of worlds were verbally express during that time as we both felt the need to be very present with Dani. We were very aware that her boy's and husband were experiencing the same emotions that we were so we stayed in contact with them. When that doctor came through the door and said he 'FOUND THE PROBLEM" your emotions run from Oh Thank God to yes, we told you something was wrong and she wasn't just crazy you ******. There were days that I questioned if I should be encouraging her to take this high-risk surgery yet; I knew in my gut that something was wrong with her physically. It was a powerful moment in my life and we gave thanks to all that supported Dani in her journey back to life.

In the days that followed Dani received loads of love from all over the country, from her friends and family. One of the most powerful moments was when she came out of the anesthesia and I told her that they found the problem. Let me repeat that, they found the problem. She looked up at me an in that instant we both knew as she smiled and softly said "they found the problem, I knew it, I've always known it".

I stayed with Dani over the next several days while she recuperated in the hospital. With a background in nursing I was able to help make sure she was getting the best care possible.

Besides making sure Dani's medical needs were being taken care of it was important she had the support of family to be there for her every step of the way to recovery. That included the weeks and months after the takedown surgery.

18

Returning Home

The day finally came when I was ready to return home after having the takedown of my RNY gastric bypass surgery. The flight attendant helped me out of the wheelchair and to my seat on the plane. She ask what happened to me and after giving her a brief explanation she proceeded with a story about a friend of hers that was very ill after having the gastric bypass surgery. She was most interested in how I found help since her friend was in need and her doctor told her that she would just have to "live with it".

That is a phrase I have heard over and over again from people who have had problems with nowhere to go. I gladly answered her questions and gave information her friend needed to get the help she deserved. It made me feel good to help any way I could, no one should have to suffer.

The flight home was a bumpy one. At that point I was even more grateful I had stayed a couple of days before getting on the plane. The flight attendant was concerned for me and very attentive. At one point she kind of scared me when she said, "if at any point there is an emergency I will get you off first". I was grateful for the offer, but it still left me a little nervous.

It was a good thing I had taken a pain pill. The discomfort from the jostling around and thought of crashing diminished. I had gone through too much to be in a plane crash so I wasn't even going to think about it. All I wanted to do is get home to my husband and family.

The plane landed safely and I was getting more excited to see my loved ones. The flight attendant had asked the captain to call ahead for a wheelchair and it was there for me when I departed the plane. My husband and one of our sons were allowed to bypass security and meet me at the gate. We picked up my luggage and went to the car.

It was a great homecoming with my husband, both our sons, and our dogs. We were so very happy to see each other again. To be in my own home and bed was just what I needed.

When I first had the gastric bypass surgery by Dr. No, I could not sleep in my bed from all the discomfort so I spent all my time a recliner chair for six weeks. This time, I went right to my bed without any problems. I also was able to get my own food prepared and take care of my needs. My husband took another couple of weeks off from work just to be with me and help if I needed it. He also took care of the household and shopping.

For the next two weeks my daily routine consisted of sleeping, taking my vitamins and minerals, eating pureed food, walking, and relaxing. After two weeks, I could add in other kinds of food which was a blessing. Nothing pureed looked appetizing, yet I followed my instructions from Dr. Compassion and the dietician. Little by little I added in a variety of foods without any problems.

It had been so long since I had food, other than broth, I was nervous about what would happen when I swallowed. To my joy, there was no pain, vomiting, or nausea. There were other physical problems that went away as well. I had no more heart palpitations, muscle and bone pain, weakness, dizziness, hair loss, dry and pale skin, back pain, high blood pressure, hypoglycemia, and depression. The thyroid medication was now also taking effect since my body was able to absorb medications as well as nutrients from food. My mood had improved so much I was able to go off of the medication for anxiety immediately after surgery. The stress of trying to get in protein and supplements to make it through a day was gone. My body was getting back into balance. I was now able to get my vitamins and minerals through food and could decrease the amount of supplements I had to take before the takedown.

My activity level increased each day, and after the six weeks the gastric tube was removed. During the six weeks with the tube in place I did develop a slight infection where the sutures were attached to my skin to make sure the tube didn't move. I was given antibiotics from my family doctor and it cleared up in a couple of days. Once the tube was removed I could then start taking showers and baths. I would not miss washing my hair and bathing from a sink, or wrapping my stomach with plastic wrap to take a shower so the gastric tube wouldn't get wet. I could now take a bath and go swimming.

I went to a surgical specialist in the area were I live to have the gastric tube removed instead of having to travel again back to Dr. Compassion's office. This gastric specialist will be the one who will do my future check-ups. He, like all the other associates in his office, will not do the gastric bypass surgery or any other WLS. After researching the pros and cons of the surgery they decided, as a group, the risks and complications were too high and the benefits to low. The doctors in this group do see patients which have problems resulting from the surgery. Most patients see their weight loss surgeon only for the first year and then they have to find other doctors to help them. This is common. It is no surprise that doctors doing the WLS don't have accurate data on long term patients if their patients choose or have to go to other doctors for further health care. There are doctors that will follow their patients for more than one year but not all do. Each person who has the WLS needs to make sure their doctor will be there for them for years and not just for the short term. The doctor who did my RNY did tell me he would be there for me if anything should ever happen, which was mostly unlikely, but he wasn't.

It was important for me to have a follow-up doctor that supported my decision to have the gastric bypass surgery takedown. I didn't need a doctor telling me I will gain my weight all back, or that I will regret having the reversal. The gastric specialist I went to, unlike some WLS surgeons, was more concerned with my health than with me being thin. He will watch for any other problems that could arise from both of the surgeries. Adhesions are always a problem with any surgery and need to be monitored for any complications.

With the takedown surgery behind me I could now look at eating as a way to sustain my life and not looked at as a chore. I didn't have to worry every day about how I was going to get in nourishment and eat 2 ounces every one to two hours. With the chronic vomiting coming to a complete halt I could now eat every few hours. Thinking about food from the time I woke up in the morning till I went to bed was now a thing of the past.

I was only able to get in 300 calories a day before the reversal and now was getting in 700 to 900 calories without any weight gain. I don't know for sure what will happen with my weight in a couple of years or ten years from now. But, that is not where I will focus my attention. The emphasis will be on my health and physical activity, it will be a life style, not a punishment. The gastric bypass was the hardest diet I have ever been on and it was not successful. It did change my life, for the worse. If I had stayed with the gastric bypass I would have died, by reversing it, I will live.

With the added daily activity I am retraining my body to accept food and not have my body think it is in starvation mode. This isn't an easy task since I have been in malnutrition for so many months. A nutritionist told me I would most likely gain some weight before maintaining because my body is starved for food. I will have to gradually add in food and increase exercising to find the balance that works for me.

Calories taken in and calories expended through exercise equates to energy in and energy out. That is the balanced way to long term control of weight. Making sure that exercising isn't done because you have to but rather because it makes you feel good will have long lasting results. Exercising works for me now when it didn't before because my attitude about it has changed. Before, I was looking at exercising more as a punishment for eating. Now, I look at exercising as a way to feel good about all aspects of my self.

Is it fair to not be able to eat more than 700 to 900 calories a day without gaining weight? – NO. I have made a choice not to count the calories I eat everyday. I decided for myself to strengthen my muscles and to eat what allows me to have a healthy body. Everyone needs to find what works best for them.

A person's metabolism can be increased by adding an exercise program without any WLS. In fact, after having WLS your metabolism will be lower than it's ever been due to chronic starvation, and that means you might not be able to eat more than 700 calories a day without gaining weight. While some WLS patients will continue to lose weight after two years others stop at six month. I stopped losing at 10 months out from the surgery, even at 300 calories a day. My metabolism had slowed down considerably.

According to my weight trainer, "if you take an approach of a low fat diet and daily exercise method of weight loss, your metabolism will be higher than it's ever been due to muscle forming, and that means you can eat more without gaining your weight back".

I probably won't be able to go up to 1,500 calories a day like I did before when I gained so much weight, but I won't rule it out. With the added exercise it is possible to add more calories without weight gain. It was never about becoming a thin person, but to have a better quality of life.

The gastric bypass surgery didn't give me a healthier life or a better quality of life, rather a much poorer one. I now know my life has been improved by having the takedown and would have it again without hesitation.

Two months after having the gastric bypass takedown my life has been wonderful. I had expected the healing from the surgery to take several weeks or months, but it was much faster than I anticipated. After eighteen months of misery, I had almost forgotten how good it feels to be well and full of energy. Eating food gave me strength and not pain or discomfort. I was able to hike two to three hours every day into the mountains by my home and go lap swimming at the recreational center. My life with my husband and children was back to normal. I could now go places with them instead of staying home due to a lack of energy or worrying about throwing up. There have been no complications from the takedown and my body was working normally.

Three months after having the takedown, my weight did increase a few pounds. The daily work-outs are firming my muscles and muscle weighs more than fat. Rapid weight loss not only causes a high amount of stress on the bodies organs, but it also causes the skin to sag. Weight training and exercise, along with a slow rate of weight loss, allows the body to tighten up gradually. The WLS is so appealing when you see people drop weight so fast. Many of us overweight people want to just wake up one morning and look into the mirror and see a thin person. Patience is a virtue and when we are willing to take the time to change the pattern in our lives that got us to where we are with our weight than we can change the pattern to take an approach that is long term and healthy.

I never did reach my target weight Dr. No said I should obtain through the gastric bypass surgery, despite the fact that the ring prevented solid food from entering my stomach which led to malnutrition. I could care less about what some chart says I should weigh. This is my body and I am comfortable with how I feel rather than how I look. According to the weight charts, I am still overweight, but my health is good and my life is full of happiness rather than the pain I had with the WLS.

There is another topic I would like to bring up regarding weight loss and weight gain that can shed some light as to why we gain so easily.

For thousands of years humans have gone through times of feast and famine. In our genetic make-up, our bodies are programmed to put on weight when food is plentiful in preparation for the times our bodies go through famines. In many countries this cycle still occurs, but in the United States most people living today haven't gone through a period of famine. Our bodies are still preparing for a time of lack of food which is not happening. Instead, every fast food establishment is super sizing the portions, and people don't feel they are getting their monies worth in restaurants if they don't have large amounts of food on their plates. A nutritionist I spoke with said, "The fat content is higher than ever before and our bodies are not able to adapt to the increase without weight gain".

In some countries, having a robust figure is a plus since that person is more likely to withstand an illness or die from starvation. A thin person is less likely to survive, leaving children without a mother or father. Men from these countries would rather have a heavier wife than a thin one; she will be more likely to be around during a time of famine or disaster. Not all societies look at overweight people as ugly and undesirable. Either I need to move to another country or deal with the one I live in.

I am not saying we should be overweight, but rather physically fit. There are thin people who don't exercise and do not have a longer life span than people who are overweight and active. It all comes down to fitness, mentally and physically.

In the United States and other countries being overweight is something to be concerned about. Especially since there are reports stating people in the United States are getting heavier every year. Excess weight can cause physical health issues and needs to be addressed between the person and their doctor. Whether weight issues are genetic, environmental, or a combination of both WLS is not the only answer to resolve being overweight.

I will continue to follow a life style, not a diet, which will enhance my quality of life. This will always include daily exercising as well as watching what I eat and why I eat. I look forward to joining others on hikes, biking, swimming, and anything else I want to do. If I hadn't had the takedown I would have been on the sidelines with a deteriorating health, never joining my family and friends in any activity.

I have never enjoyed fast food or fatty foods so it is easy for me to continue to avoid those types of food. I will stay with the types of food I ate before the RNY but smaller amounts. I know I do not require many calories and deal with it. Even with a few pounds of weight gain I am now stronger, have more endurance, and am so much healthier.

19

Expenses

The expenses I have incurred from all the problems from the RNY surgery during the last year and a half have been astronomical. The total cost is well over $100,000 for the original WLS, drugs, supplements, therapy, time taken off of work to take care of me, having my twin sister fly to my home for two weeks to make sure I got in food during a severe depression, flights for a consultation in another state, a trip for testing, then the trip for the reversal, hotels, and car rentals, lost income from my business when I had to stop working and much more. It would have been cheaper and less painful to hire a personal trainer and a chef. Although I am feeling better and don't anticipate any further problems, the follow-up expenses have continued. I still have to deal with the lack of a strong immune system because the surgery depleted my body of nutrients for so long. It will take time to rebuild my body and get it strong again.

I sold off most of my business inventory to help defray the costs and used money from our family savings. It bothered me greatly to take money meant for our son's college education to pay for medical expenses. We discussed this as a family and they were more than willing to use the money if it meant I would be able to live.

I figured it was not worth having a business inventory if I could no longer continue with my business so that was an easy decision. My insurance company covered much of the direct medical expenses. We were responsible for 30% of the reversal, all of the travel expenses, going to the naturopath, plus all the supplements, during the eighteen months with the RNY.

Several people interviewed stated they have spent over $600,000 which their insurance company did not pay all of the expenses. One woman's insurance company didn't pay for most of her expenses. She had over $200,000 in medical expenses during a seven year period she was responsible for. This woman is still sick and continues to add to the amount of money she already owes. Emergency room expenses, hospital stays, medications, doctors visits, surgeries, all add up and are overwhelming when insurance companies won't cover all the charges. There is also a matter of losing your insurance if you can no longer hold down a job. Some insurance companies won't pay for follow-up care after the WLS. It is up to the patient to pay out of pocket for these expenses. Some people end up in bankruptcy when they can no longer pay the bills or won't see their doctor because they can't pay out of pocket for tests or surgeries.

It is easier for doctors to get the gastric bypass surgery approved through the insurance company's than it is to get the takedown. Those that I have heard from who had the takedown went through many tests to prove to the insurance company that they were sick enough to warrant the takedown. I have been told that if a patient wants to pay for the reversal 'out of pocket' it is easier to get a doctor to do the procedure.

Once the insurance companies start having to pay out more for the takedowns they will start re-evaluating the initial gastric bypass surgery. I have read that some major hospitals and insurance companies are now stopping the approval for the gastric bypass surgery.

For example: There was an article on www.obesityhelp.org in June of 2002 stating a hospital in Texas is putting a hold on their bariatric program. The article said, "Finances did not play a part in this. We are not planning on eliminating our bariatric program. However, we are putting it on hold. Due to the high volume of cases we are seeing and since this is still considered a new program, this is part of our normal review process." The article said it wasn't about money, even though the weight loss surgeries do bring in a great deal of money. The hospital didn't say if they were being sued or had concerns about the long term problems patients are having with these surgeries. Time will only tell why some hospitals are putting a hold on their bariatric programs. To the thousands of us who have and still do have problems, it doesn't surprise us.

Money being paid out for long term medical problems from the gastric bypass surgery is likely to go up rather than down. We all know how difficult it can be to get insurance companies to cover medical expenses, and if they start losing a great deal of money they will take a look at whether to cover this procedure and then pay again for takedowns.

Medical expenses can be added up, but emotional ones cannot. I would never wish what I have gone through on anyone. Family and friends are so important for support. But, what has made a great deal of difference in my life is talking with others who have gone through what I have. We have something in common that can't always be put into words. It is like trying to explain to a woman who has never had a baby what it is like going through childbirth. *Unless one goes through the experience first hand it is difficult to fully comprehend the magnitude of what it is like to have problems with the gastric bypass surgery.*

There is help for those that want their life and their health back and are having life threatening medical problems with the gastric bypass surgery. It may take a great deal of determination to find the right support team to walk with you through the journey to a healthier life. I didn't want to "*just live with it*" like I have been told by those in the on-line support groups that did not want to hear about any problems and were against having the takedown. I chose not to live as an invalid, but rather to regain control of my health and life. I have more work to do here on Mother Earth and want to live a life of joy!

20

Stories from Others

Once I lowered my wall of protection and was willing to put myself out there to let others know about having the gastric bypass surgery, the stories started coming in. Hundreds of them!

These are just a few examples of experiences other's have had with their gastric bypass surgery. I wish that all the personal life experiences I have run across were happy and with a positive outcome, but that is not the case. The following are just a few of the stories I have been told, and there are many, many, more.

Annie's Story

Annie did not have the WLS, but her input is valuable so I included it in this section, as well as the stories from those who had the surgery.

I met Annie at a Holistic Fair that we both participated in (prior to my WLS reversal). She showed me the Body Balance products by Life Force she represents and I read all her material and decided to try them. After talking for awhile I told her I had the gastric bypass surgery and she thought these products would be beneficial. I tried them, but found I could not keep them down. I vomited them out so they were not meant for me. Then again, I vomited everything so it wasn't the product, it was me. I have given them to my family which has been very helpful.

Annie is from England and told me she had firsthand knowledge about the Roux-en-Y gastric bypass reversals. She had worked at a hospital where all these surgeries were routinely reversed after twelve to eighteen months. She did not know if all the hospitals in England did the reversals, only the one she worked at. This was most interesting since all I kept hearing is that they are not reversible. Annie said there is a department in the hospital where she worked that was set up just for the reversals. I asked Annie to get me as much information as she could regarding the reversal, why they reverse them, and what the patient goes through to be qualified to have the gastric bypass in the first place.

After a couple of weeks Annie got back to me with the information. Her father and brother are doctors in

England and they were able to contact another doctor who had knowledge of the reversals. In England they have much higher guidelines for those seeking the gastric bypass surgery than in the United States. People in England that do not qualify are coming to the United States.

Patients in England know it will be reversed when they go into it. After the procedure they are worked with much more closely than in the United States. The reason why they reverse them is due to long term complications from malnutrition and mal-absorption. This surgery was meant to help those who are severely morbidly obese to reduce their weight and once that is achieved the surgery is reversed to prevent long term health problems. A person cannot stay in malnutrition and mal-absorption for life without long term affects.

Annie was shocked to learn that patients in the United States were not having the WLS reversed automatically. She was also amazed at how many WLS were being performed on people who would not qualify in England. It appears WLS is being done on more people in the United States for cosmetic reasons rather than health reasons.

This story is not meant to scare people or to have everyone running to their doctor's to inquire about the gastric bypass reversal, nor, if they should be getting this done. I feel it is important for everyone considering the bypass surgery to look into all aspects of it before making a decision to have this procedure. Arming yourself with information can only help with the decision. Those that have already had a weight loss surgery need to be monitored for long term complications.

Annie continues to be of great support for me and she will provide nutritional advice. She is one of those rare people who have great empathy and compassion for others. Annie wants to help and does in so many ways. We all need the support from family and friends and I was very lucky to have her come into my life when I needed help. Her expertise about the reversal helped me get the answers I was seeking and gave me the encouragement to move forward.

Sandy's Story

One evening I got a call from a man, I will call Tom and his wife Sandy. Tom got my phone number through a call list from Dr. No's office.

I did not know why my name was on the call list because I never gave permission.

Tom was calling me for his wife, Sandy, since she is just as private a person as I am and she was very ill. Sandy was in such pain that she did not want to talk to anyone at that point. Tom asked me about my experience with Dr. No and the Roux-en-Y surgery. At first I was hesitant about discussing anything since I did not know this person.

After talking with Tom for several minutes I realized he was in search of someone that had been having problems and could relate with his wife. Tom told me they had called several people on the calling list from Dr. No's office and *felt they were not being honest with them.*

Tom stated that he was so relieved to finally find someone that was willing to admit they had problems with this surgery. Like me, he also found people on the calling list were not honest with him, and others were reluctant to say anything about their problems.

Tom described what Sandy had gone through since the day she had her surgery to the present. Her story and what she was going through just broke my heart. After that initial conversation with Tom, Sandy felt comfortable talking with me directly. We have had many talks and continue to keep in contact with each other.

From the time Sandy awoke from her surgery to the time she got her gastric bypass reversal, which was a long seven months, she had been on high dosages of pain medication just so she could get in 200 calories a day. Her weight had been dropping very rapidly and her life consisted of staying in bed or sitting in a chair. Sandy cried daily as her health deteriorated further with every passing day. Tom had to take care of her, his business, and their children.

Sandy had undergone tests, but they were inconclusive as to what was causing her pain. She knew that she could not live a life in bed and on the strong drugs just so she could get in a small amount of food. Dr. No continued to refuse to perform a reversal even though he had no answers for her deteriorating condition. Sandy and Tom finally threatened Dr. No with a lawsuit in order to get him to agree to perform the reversal.

After seven months, Sandy finally got her gastric bypass reversed (takedown). The cause for Sandy's intense pain was thought to be a cut nerve from the original surgery. There was no sure answer as to why she ended up in such pain. Her pouch was full of ulcers so it had to be taken away before reconnecting her original stomach. Sandy was informed by the surgical nurse that when she was opened up the original surgery had not healed. The endoscope procedure failed to detect this.

I am glad to tell you Sandy is now doing wonderfully and has regained her health. Sandy kept losing weight for seven months after the reversal and then stabilized. After a year she has gained back ten pounds but it healthy and active again with her family. She was told it would all come back immediately, but that never happened.

Sandy was prepared for some weight gain and it wouldn't have bothered her. Weight loss was secondary to having a quality life. Now she has her health back and is happy and with no regrets having the reversal.

Brad's Story

This is a short story that I feel is important because if Brad would have had the help he deserved the end results may have turned out differently.

Blood tests are one way a doctor can tell how their patients are doing, but they also need to listen to the patient. Patients know when they do not feel right and this should be respected just as much, or more, than tests.

A friend of mine in another state knew of my circumstance with the gastric bypass and thought I might be able to help Brad, even if it was just to talk with him. Brad had been losing weight very fast following his WLS, and had several problems. His blood work up kept showed nothing out of the ordinary so he continued with the program.

Within two months of his previous blood work-up, which was within the normal range, a second blood work-up gave results that were alarming.

Efforts were made to help him but it was too late. Brad's health did not improve. It only got worse over time and he passed on. *Brad died of starvation, his heart and organs could not take the malnutrition any longer and his body gave out.*

I never got a chance to talk with Brad. He died before my friend could give him my phone number and this saddens me a great deal. He was trying to save his life by having the surgery and ended up dying a slow death.

Debby's Story

Debby had been looking into having the WLS and was concerned whether it was the right choice for her. She had difficulty walking because of her weight and talked with her family physician about the surgery.

She had a bone density test to make sure she wasn't having a problem with osteoporosis. The bone tests showed she had no deterioration of her bones. One of the problems patients with the WLS have is osteoporosis because of an inability to absorb calcium. This test was important for her to have checked out before going through surgery because of the pain she was having in her legs.

Debby wanted to know about the pros and cons of the different types of surgeries being performed. Like most people researching the WLS she found wonderful stories about it and not much else. She thought, like most of us who went through with the surgery, she had all the information needed to make an informed decision and proceeded with the WLS.

The doctor Debby went to for the gastric bypass surgery did the RNY/Fobi form of the WLS. She asked many questions, especially about being able to walk with ease if the weight were off. The doctor told her *she would be able to not only walk, but would be able to go jogging once she lost her weight.* He was reassuring the problems of walking would go away and that the risks of complications were minimal.

Debby had no complications after her surgery and went home, ready to lose the weight, and begin walking to places she had only dreamed about. She was looking forward to taking walks with her grandchildren and husband.

The first year went by, and then the second year without any major problems and she had lost weight. She was taking all of her vitamins, minerals, and calcium. Debby had thought the surgery was the best thing she ever did until everything started going down hill.

While walking one day, she fell down and broke her leg. She was in a cast for weeks and after the cast was off she started physical therapy to get mobility back. A couple of weeks later she fell again and broke her other leg. Again, she was in a cast for weeks and more weeks of recovery. Her bones were not breaking from the fall. *Rather, she was falling because her bones were breaking.*

Breaking two legs in a short period of time sent a signal to her and her family doctor that something wasn't going right. A bone density scan was performed and her bones were deteriorating very rapidly. Debby's doctor wanted to monitor her for the next several months and had her increase her calcium intake.

Over the next year Debby had broken the bones in her legs several more times. Before further bone breakage, her doctor recommended surgery to strengthen her legs. Steel rods were placed in her legs for reinforcement. Debby spent months recovering from this surgery and now is just beginning to walk again with the help of a walker. Physical therapy is helping and she doesn't know yet if she will ever be able to walk on her own.

Debby is now concentrating on getting the strength needed to undergo a reversal of her gastric bypass surgery. She is at a high risk of other bones being broken due to the lack of calcium absorption into her body.

Debby had read that she would have to take calcium for life once having the WLS, but had no idea she wouldn't be able to absorb the recommended amount. She had increased the amount of calcium after the first bone broke, but that didn't prevent it from it happening again, and again.

Debby is now worse off than before having the WLS. She was told she would be able to walk and jog. Now she can't do either!

Since she is also inactive she has gained back most of her weight and is more depressed. She was told, like all of us, weight loss is permanent and like any weight loss program, you have to exercise and she is not able to do it.

From the low calorie intake for so long after having the WLS she now has ruined her metabolism and can't eat more than 1,000 calories a day without weight gain.

It's no wonder she is depressed, but Debby is now getting the help she needs. She has a great family doctor, and the support of family, friends, and therapist. The doctor that performed her WLS will not do a reversal for her and she is now trying to find help. She is hopeful everything will get better. Her optimism to wonderful and she is taking one step at a time to recovery.

Ellen's Story

Ellen was so excited about having the gastric bypass surgery, looking forward to a healthy life and a slim body. Her surgery day came and she was ready to begin a new way of living. There were no complications with the surgery and she went home from the hospital to recover and to start losing weight.

Ellen felt that if she were thinner she could do all the things slender people took for granted. She wanted to wear small sized clothing and could do this if she lost 100 pounds.

The months went by and as the pounds dropped off, Ellen was happy. She watched the amount she ate and made sure the food was healthy. It had been almost two years since Ellen had the gastric bypass surgery and she felt she was one of the success stories, but that was about to change.

One morning she woke up and had pain in her stomach so she went to the hospital. They examined her and sent her home, saying "there is nothing wrong with you". Ellen went home.

Later that same day Ellen returned to the hospital complaining of the same problems. The pain had gotten worse and she didn't want to go home this time without an answer. Again, they checked her out, said everything was fine and sent her home.

That evening Ellen went back to the hospital after throwing up "stool from her bowels". This time they knew she was very ill and did surgery on her immediately. Ellen's stomach had burst and toxins had spread throughout her entire body.

Surgeons removed the burst stomach and did the reversal in hopes of saving her life. *Ellen was in a coma for two months in the intensive care unit at the hospital.* She was fighting for her life, and would eventually win.

Ellen stayed in the hospital five months recovering from the ordeal. She never knew for sure why her pouch burst. It might have been from adding in a small amount of food or another reason.

Some patients with the gastric bypass surgery can tolerate more than two ounces of food because the stomach may stretch. Yet, others can have their stomach burst. Usually, a patient will throw up if their stomach is too full, but not always. In Ellen's case the stomach burst and she almost died.

Ellen's weight had dropped under a hundred pounds from being so sick from her gastric bypass surgery. She regrets the day she ever heard about the surgery and would never recommend it to anyone. The risk she took almost cost her everything. Being thin and able to wear smaller clothes was not worth what she went through.

Life for Ellen is getting better now that she has had the reversal and the doctor's were able to do the necessary repairs. She takes it one day at a time and is putting her energy into getting well.

Mary's Story

The following on-line letter was written by Mary (with an underlined edit for clarity):

My name is Mary and I am a 17 year post-op VBG victim. I am one of the veterans of WLS nobody can find (or wants to find). Almost from the get-go after having WLS I began to throw up and have abdominal pain. And for16 years I have been hiding in bathrooms in public places waiting for patrons to leave so I could throw up. In October of 2000 I began to have severe pain in abdominal area. I had a nice job at a school cafeteria, but had to quit because of my medical problems. I must have seen a dozen doctors before I finally found a GP DR, i.e., general practitioner doctor, who would help me find a gastroenterologist willing to help me. I guess WLS victims are "hot potatoes" every doctor I went to would not try to help me because of the risk of bleeding to death, etc.

I was in chronic pain for 6 months. And it seems to people who are fortunate enough to have thin cells instead of fat cells, think obese people do not get sick. After 10 years I weighed about 200 and still could not eat over 2 oz. Finally the gastroenterologist did a stomach scope and stretched my band and put me on meds for chronic pain and I am 100% better. I have gained 75 lbs in 6 months... but I am pain free. But only if I take this medicine. I will always have a mutant stomach because after X amount of years, the stomach tissue and hernia wrap around the staple; and no-one can even see the whole VBG. I had many procedures and tests too numerous to name, before I found the right doctor.

I was a member with the Obesity Chat line when I was in so much pain. The majority of them attacked me accusing me of sabotage.

Which is far from the truth, rather I gave support to the post-ops and the pre-ops. I was desperate to find a good doctor. All the specialists who perform WLS would not help me or even discuss my options (except to encourage me to have a revision). If I had known what I do now; it is a toss up if I would have had WLS. I got it done in the pioneer days when it and the intestinal bypass were new. I want to share my story with whoever is considering WLS.

Sincerely, Mary

The following are additional letters from Mary since she wrote the above letter:

On late term leaks and the condition of her stomach, 18 years after surgery:

> I think in regards to late term leaks...sometimes even with all the tests and procedures they zing in on a certain thing (like a hernia for example) and do not observe anything else. I had a stomach scope from one Doc who told my husband "everything is ok... I knew I wouldn't be able to see anything anyway." Then in the surgery room I heard him tell another Doc, "see what a mess this stomach and hernia are in" So there goes a $2,000 procedure for no advice...no diagnosis, but from I would say an ambitious Doc. So after a dozen Docs another one operated on me thru the throat and stretched my vertical band out. He said, "I don't see even how you could have eaten anything your stomach looks like an

hourglass. Not to mention scar tissue, hiatal hernia, and appendages.

On gas after surgery:

> WLS patients have a lot of gas because when your tummy is operated on gas is trapped in body for X amount of time. The best thing to do is walk it off and try to belch. I know that sounds gross) but this will help you. Also I read someone talking about a reversal. If you have had your surgery over 2 years you cannot get a reversal. They can't even see my staples, they are covered with hernia and stomach mass. And, your doctor will have to be honest and tell u this is true. When they do a revision the tummy is re-stapled over old surgery.

> It is heartbreaking to me that being a person of size makes a lot of us feel humiliated, like we are bad people because we are of size. Anyway whomever decides to go ahead and get WLS I wish u much success and happiness.

> The thing about WLS that is upsetting is how someone can determine long lasting results in 2 years...

> Sincerely, Mary

April 12.2002:

> I have wanted to ask you something. I would like to participate in an obesity research program. I am desperate about my continuous weight gain still only can eat 3 oz. But I am re-

living the pain and humiliation I suffered so long in my childhood and as a young adult. I don't want to leave the house for fear of ridicule. This presents problems for my husband and daughter and me. I am trying not to eat high caloric foods. Also I have Lupus, osteoporosis and dropped bladder and bowel. And there is speculation that my WLS could have created these physical ailments.

April 12, 2002:

And my doctor says I will have to have my [silastic] band stretched out once a year. It has been about 8 months since this was done and the last 3 weeks I am still throwing up and gaining weight. But I am lucky to have a competent specialist.

On regain and aftermath: April 26, 2002

I personally know 5 post-ops that are at least 15 years in. 2 of my friends have died on the table getting WLS; 2 have gained all their weight back and more. And the 5th is like me suffering and up to her butt with lots of med problems due to WLS. Does everyone assume all veteran WLS patients have computers? You think they are standing in line to brag about how they are heavier than when they had surgery. With all the bigotry and self-esteem problems people who are of size have had...this doesn't seem logical to anyone.

Being an obese person is so painful in many ways no wonder we are all willing to let the Docs cut us up with no fear of the

future. There are a couple of WLS veterans here in this club that says they doing well and that is great. I would in no way wish the heartache, med bills, loss of jobs from being sick; and the humiliation of gaining all our weight back after spending thousands of dollars to try and lose weight. I am happy for anyone who is doing well; but the only people post-ops who can give a valid opinion are veteran post-ops.

On would she have the surgery again - April 29th, 2002

Personally, I (in retrospect) would much rather pass away as a person of size before my time (and lots of obese folks live to be old) than to go thru what I have been thru and probably will have to file bankruptcy after all this post-op care. For the rest of my life. Some Docs do use scare tactics...as some preachers do too (going to hell......etc.) I am 44 years old I want to have fun and be a normal wife and mother. I am trapped in this body. Not a thin person crying to get out! But... want to be a regular person.

Laura's Story

Well here's a condensed version in Laura's own words (bms stands for bowels movements)...

Heard about WLS, was excited about WLS, had WLS, nearly died, wanted to die, lost 60-70#

because of WLS... Had diarrhea, 20+ bms a day [author's note: BMs stands for Bowel Movements], gas like barn yard animal smell, vitamin mineral depletions, lost half my hair, soft nails, pasty white skin, yellowed whites of my eyes, acne pustules, pimples all over my face, complete loss of energy at different times, stomach distention, pseudo bowel obstructions, hernias, adhesions, hemorrhoids, nausea for 10 years straight (and many other things I want to forget)... lost down to a size 6 five years later with depression, gained back up to 240# a year later(started out at 297#)... Was getting divorced and knew my good BCBS [author's note: BCBS stands for **B**lue **C**ross® **B**lue **S**hield®] would be cancelled. So got JIB reversed and here I am.......None the thinner or healthier for doing all that.

21

Comparison of WLS

Procedures

The tables in this chapter provide a comparison of the following types of weight loss surgeries currently performed, provided by Sue Widemark.

- Adjustable Lap Band, AGB
- Duodenal Switch, BPD-DS,
- Distal Gastric Bypass with DS
- RNY, Gastric Bypass, Roux-en-Y, LAP, RNY
- Vertical Banded Gastroplasty (VBG)

The following topics are addressed for each type of surgery.

- How It Works
- What It Does
- How Is It Done

- Long Term Weight Loss Success
- Recovery Time
- Complications - Short Term
- Complications - Long Term
- Is It Reversible
- Long Term Dietary Modifications
- Nutritional Supplement
- Have To Exercise To Keep Or Maintain Weight Loss
- Lifespan
- How Long Has It Been Done

Factor	Vertical Banded Gastro-plasty (VBG)	RNY, Gastric Bypass, Roux-en-Y, LAP, RNY	Duodenal Switch, BPD-DS, Distal Gastric Bypass with DS	Adjustable Lap Band, AGB
How It Works	Restricts amount of food intake at meals	Restricts amounts of food + Malabsorptive + doesn't absorb some nutrients	Slightly Restrictive but very Malabsorptive + doesn't absorb or digest MOST nutrients	Restricts amount of food intake at meals
What It Does	Causes a situation of low cal diet and bulimia	Very low cal diet with poor absorption of fats and protein + about 300 to 700 calories a day, first year + some bulimia	Same as gastric bypass but less absorption of nutrients. Bulimia only through the gut i.e. diarrhea (some patients do vomit but not as much as with the RNY)	Low cal diet about 1000 to 1500 calories a day unless patient "cheats" surgery

Factor	Vertical Banded Gastro-plasty (VBG)	RNY, Gastric Bypass, Roux-en-Y, LAP, RNY	Duodenal Switch, BPD-DS, Distal Gastric Bypass with DS	Adjustable Lap Band, AGB
How Is It Done	Stomach is stapled so that it's in two parts, an upper pouch and the rest. A hole in the stomach separates the two parts and a hard silastic ring is placed around the opening of the pouch into the main stomach.	Stomach is stapled and divided into two parts, the 1 or 2 oz "pouch" and the larger part which is bypassed. The top part of the small gut is also bypassed (18 inches to 6 feet). The top part of the gut - bypassed - is where you digest vitamins and absorb a lot of food.	Stomach is divided and separated into two parts, stapled lengthwise (retaining the lower stomach valve). The pouch part is 4-5 oz. The 36 oz part of the stomach not a part of the pouch is discarded (removed from the body). The top of the small gut (about 2 inches) is left attached to the tiny pouch. Then, the small bowel is cut into two pieces and rearranged so that 60 percent of it is bypassed. The pouch part is reattached to the last segment of small gut (or part thereof), leaving about 2.5 feet of small gut where food goes which is usually called "the common tract" Digestive juices are supposed to meet food in common tract but most are re-absorbed in traveling through long section of bypassed gut (see Scopinaro and Hess reports). In this surgery, the gall bladder and appendix are removed at the time of original surgery.	A silicon ring is placed at the top of the stomach to create a roadblock for food passing quickly. No stomach stapling involved and no intestinal bypass. The ring lies outside the stomach and has a soft inner bag which is filled with saline (to adjust size of opening into stomach) with a lead placed usually under the ribcage.

Factor	Vertical Banded Gastroplasty (VBG)	RNY, Gastric Bypass, Roux-en-Y, LAP, RNY	Duodenal Switch, BPD-DS, Distal Gastric Bypass with DS	Adjustable Lap Band, AGB
Long Term Weight Loss Success	Poor Most patients appear to re-gain with this surgery. The type of foods that can be comfortably eaten are high fat and not nutritious. Veggies, meats extremely difficult to eat	Average 70% maintain some weight loss, 25 percent gain it all back (see Hebrew University Study, 1999)	Above Average Despite the fact the intestinal bypass of this surgery has been done for 25 years, only a handful of over 19 year patients are available + Scopinaro listed about 150 pts most of who had kept most of their weight off.	Average 70% maintain some weight loss, 25 percent gain it all back (same as gastric bypass + see the Miller study of 900 patients)
Recovery Time	1-2 days in hospital, 6 weeks recovery	1-5 days in hospital if no complications, several weeks recovery	1-5 days in hospital, if no complications + 3 months recovery	1 to 2 days hospital, 1 to 3 weeks recovery

Factor	Vertical Banded Gastro-plasty (VBG)	RNY, Gastric Bypass, Roux-en-Y, LAP, RNY	Duodenal Switch, BPD-DS, Distal Gastric Bypass with DS	Adjustable Lap Band, AGB
Compli-cations - Short Term	Vomiting, heartburn, blocking of opening to larger stomach.	Vomiting and nausea, plugging of the openings from the pouch to the small gut, poor absorption of fat soluble vitamins, E, K, A, and D, narrowing of the openings from the pouch to the small gut and where the bypassed small gut is reconnected, bowel obstruction, hernia (even with lap surgery), intestinal and pouch ulcers and or rotting, dumping syndrome (bad reaction to carbs intake), protein deficiency, ketosis (body consumes itself for proteins etc), staples coming out causing leakage of digestive juices and possible peritonitis (peritonitis can cause multiple disabilities), heart damage from rapid weight loss and/or from surgical complications, damage to organs surrounding surgical field (especially in lap procedures).	Same as gastric bypass except, most do not have dumping syndrome, less ulceration of small gut, no narrowing of stomach opening (bottom stomach valve still in place), less vomiting. In addition to complications seen with gastric bypass, the following can occur: severe protein starvation (see Scopinaro report), very foul smelling diarrhea, anemia.	Vomiting, heartburn, blocking of opening to larger stomach, lack of weight loss (some patients can easily eat around this surgery), swelling of stomach if body tries to reject the band probably requires re-surgery.

Factor	Vertical Banded Gastro-plasty (VBG)	RNY, Gastric Bypass, Roux-en-Y, LAP, RNY	Duodenal Switch, BPD-DS, Distal Gastric Bypass with DS	Adjustable Lap Band, AGB
Compli cations - Long Term	Autoimmu ne disease can occur if patients don't take liquid supplement s - apparently patients tend to stay away from nutritious foods due to difficulty in eating them, teeth rotting from vomiting (longer term patients have this), adhesions blocking opening to pouch requiring surgery. Adhesions covering stomach where stapled	Vomiting and nausea, tooth rotting from vomiting, esophagus problems from vomiting, autoimmune disease (probably from B12 shortage), osteoporosis (brittle porous bones) from inability to digest calcium, adhesions blocking openings to small gut, ulcers, bowel obstruction, micronutrient deficiencies (like zinc etc), fat soluble vitamin deficiency, A, E, K and D (causing night blindness etc), pernicious anemia (from B12 deficiency), iron poor anemia, immune system breakdown, organ shutdown, kidney stones, liver damage, and early death (see ASBS.org complications on ANY surgery involving malabsorption)	General malnutrition (regardless of supplementation) causing brain damage etc, osteoporosis, protein malnutrition disease, autoimmune disease, Sjogrens Syndrome (drying of mucus tissues in body), severe anemia, poor absorption and digestion of fat soluble vitamins, A, E, D, K, causing night blindness etc, immune system breakdown, diarrhea, narrowing of small gut, bowel obstruction, organ shutdown, kidney stones, liver damage, and early death (see ASBS list of complications on JIB intestinal bypass. The BPD done with this surgery is a variation of the JIB)	Slippage of band, infection on outside of stomach (requiring removal of band), breakage of lead to fill band, blockage of opening between pouch and stomach, esophagal damage and ulcers. Some American doctors are charging for fills - adjustment s ($150 per fill)

Factor	Vertical Banded Gastro-plasty (VBG)	RNY, Gastric Bypass, Roux-en-Y, LAP, RNY	Duodenal Switch, BPD-DS, Distal Gastric Bypass with DS	Adjustable Lap Band, AGB
Is It Revers-ible?	Not really. If patient seeks reversal in the first couple of years after surgery, they can remove the silastic ring which gives the patient some relief from the narrowing of the opening.	Partially. A hole is made in the bypassed stomach and the small pouch is attached to the hole which reconnects the greater stomach and the duodenum or top of the small gut. Patients still suffer repercussions and often reversal surgery includes hours of removing adhesions from the stomach and removing parts of the small gut which have rotted.	The DS/BPD is not only NOT reversible but basically has no exit route except reconnecting parts of the small gut which have not rotted.	Totally reversible.

Factor	Vertical Banded Gastro-plasty (VBG)	RNY, Gastric Bypass, Roux-en-Y, LAP, RNY	Duodenal Switch, BPD-DS, Distal Gastric Bypass with DS	Adjustable Lap Band, AGB
Long Term Dietary Modifi-cation	Extremely poor diet-Patients have difficulty consuming nutritious food since it plugs the opening at the silastic ring.	After a year or two, most patients can eat most foods even sweets but have to restrict intake and exercise because they tend to regain easily. Many of them join Weight Watchers or Jenny Craig	This surgery "works" the longest of all but at about the 7 year point or so, patient must start restricting food intake and exercise or regains. Fatty food tends to cause more diarrheas.	Can eat a normal diet which means have to DIET and exercise or little to no weight is lost.
Nutri-tional Supple-ment	Multi vitamin, Iron, Calcium For life, possibly B12 shots	Protein drinks (protein poorly digested), B12 shots once or twice a week (NECESSARY), sub lingual iron, calcium citrate (not known how much calcium patients can absorb - too much calcium not used ends up in the kidneys as stones)	Protein drinks, calcium citrate (see gastric bypass note on absorption), Possibly B12 shots, sub lingual iron + SHOULD BE CLOSELY MONITORED by gastroenterologist for LIFETIME	Same as normal. (digestive system is not changed in this surgery)

Factor	Vertical Banded Gastro-plasty (VBG)	RNY, Gastric Bypass, Roux-en-Y, LAP, RNY	Duodenal Switch, BPD-DS, Distal Gastric Bypass with DS	Adjustable Lap Band, AGB
Have To Exercise To Keep Or Maintain Weight Loss?	Yes	Yes	Yes, but can avoid exercise for a few years until surgery stops "working"	Yes
How Long Has It Been Done	Since 1980 + invented by Mason to overcome nutritional problems with the gastric bypass (also his invention)	Since 1965 + a variation of the Billroth II invented in 1898 for saving lives of patients with upper small gut ulcers	BPD: 1975 (intestinal bypass part) DS (stomach part) since early 1990's	Since 1993
Lifespan	Unknown + many patients still alive at the 20 year point	Unknown. Statistics have not been released (despite surgery having been done for 40 years) and death statistics are incorrect because most gastric bypass deaths are recorded as from other causes.	Unknown. No statistics on this have been released.	Normal (in Miller study of 900 patients over 9 years, no deaths were recorded in study participants - 98 percent follow-up)

The following are several medical articles which are technical, do not include a lot of long-term follow-up advice, and may be more of a use to physicians:

Balsiger BM, Poggio JL, Mai J, Kelly KA, Sarr MG, Ten and more years after vertical banded gastroplasty as primary operation for morbid obesity, Gastrointestinal Surgery 2000 Nov-Dec;4(6):598-605.

Balsiger BM et all, Prospective evaluation of Roux-en-Y gastric bypass as primary operation for medically complicated obesity. Mayo Clinic proc. 2000 Jul; 75(7):669-72.

Oh CH, Kim HJ, Oh S, Weight loss following transected gastric bypass with proximal Roux-en-Y, Obesity Surgery 1997 Apr;7(2):142.

Reinhold Rb, Late results of gastric bypass surgery for morbid obesity, J Am College Nutrition 1994 Aug;13(4):326-31.

Avinoah E et all, [Long-term weight changes after Roux-en-Y gastric bypass for morbid obesity]. Harefuah 1993 Feb 15; 124(4):185-7,248.

Brolin RE et all, Lipid Risk profile and weight stability after gastric restrictive operations for morbid obesity, J Gastrointestinal Surgery 2000 Sep-Oct;4(5):464-9.

Scopinaro N; Adami GF; Marinari GM; Gianetta E; Traverso E; Friedman D; Camerini G; Baschieri G; Simonelli A, Biliopancreatic diversion, World J Surgery 1998 Sep;22(9):936-46.

Hess DS; Hess DW, Biliopancreatic diversion with a duodenal switch, Obesity Surgery 1998 Jun;8(3):267-82.

Baltasar A; Bou R; Bengochea M; Arlandis F; Escriva C; Mir J; Martinez R; Perez N, Duodenal switch: an effective therapy for morbid obesity--intermediate results, Obesity Surgery 2001 Feb;11(1):54-8.

Marceau P; Hould FS; Simard S; Lebel S; Bourque RA; Potvin M; Biron S, Biliopancreatic diversion with duodenal switch, World J Surgery 1998 Sep;22(9):947-54.

Marceau P; Hould FS; Potvin M; Lebel S; Biron S, Biliopancreatic diversion (duodenal switch procedure), European J Gastroenterology Hepatology 1999 Feb;11(2):99-103.

Mitchell JE, Lancaster KL, Burgard MA, Howell M, Krahn DD, Crosby RD, Wonderlich SA, Gonsell BA, Long –term Follow up of patients' Status after Gastric Bypass, Obesity Surgery, August 2001,11(4) 464-468.

Sanyal AJ, Sugerman HJ, Kellum JM, Engle KM, Wolfe L.,Stomal complications of gastric bypass: incidence and outcome of therapy, Am J Gastroenterology 1992 Sep;87(9):1165-9.

Mallory GN, Macgregor AM, Rand CS, The Influence of Dumping on Weight Loss After Gastric Restrictive Surgery for Morbid Obesity. Obesity Surgery 1996 Dec;6(6):474-478.

McLean LD, Rhode BM, Sampalis J, Forse KA Results of the surgical treatment of obesity. Am J Surgery 1993;165:155 - 59.

Avinoah E, Ovanat A, Charuzi I., Nutritional status seven years after Roux-en-Y gastric bypass surgery. Surgery 1992 Feb; 111(2):137-42.

Source: WLS surgery Center http://gastricbypass.netfirms.com/comparisonsurgery.htm

22

WLS Risk and Benefit

I am including Dr. Ernsberger's article because it provides valuable information for anyone who is assessing the pros and cons before making a decision to have a weight loss surgery.

The following article by Paul Ernsberger, Ph.D. titled "Surgery for Weight Loss: Comparison of Risk and Benefit", published from Obesity & Health (renamed Healthy Weight Journal) March-April 1991, pp. 24-25.

As the eve of the 1991 NIH consensus conference on weight loss surgery approaches, let us look back at the last NIH conference on this topic in December 1978. The panel gave its approval to intestinal bypass surgery, even though this operation was already coming under criticism for the long-term side-effects that it caused. As a result of recommendations by the consensus panel, intestinal bypass was accepted for health insurance coverage, which made possible tens of thousands of these operations. The legacy of the NIH panel's endorsement of intestinal bypass surgery is perhaps a hundred thousand patients worldwide, the majority of whom have suffered severe complications. Of the survivors, most now have had the operation undone. One can only hope that the legacy of this latest panel is more benign.

The panel members face a difficult task in evaluating the risks of the various surgical treatments for obesity. Nearly every surgical operation originates in a laboratory, where it is refined by extensive tests in animals. For example, coronary bypass surgery was the product of years of experimentation on dogs in which repeated measurements and detailed autopsies revealed potential complications and allowed surgeons to perfect the operation. In contrast, only three animal tests have ever been reported or gastric bypass or gastroplasty. In one test of gastric bypass in rats, many abnormalities were found at autopsy, including damage to the stomach, liver and pancreas from fibrosis (American Journal of Clinical Nutrition 40:293-302, 1984). We don't know whether these progressive abnormalities happen in human patients, because autopsy results have never been reported. Because of a lack of animal testing, the panelists will lack information on the biological effects of these operations.

Another difficulty the panelists will face is the bewildering variety of operations. As many as two dozen basic types of both gastroplasty and gastric bypass are in current use, along with several modifications of the original intestinal bypass. If we then consider variations on the basic methods, it can almost be said that no two surgeons do exactly the same procedure. The different types of operations differ in their safety and effectiveness. Operations such as gastric bypass that impair the absorption and processing of nutrients produce the greatest weight loss, and are most likely to produce lasting weight loss. With gastroplasty, weight regain is more common. After the most effective operation of this type, the vertical banded gastroplasty, 76% of patients failed to maintain weight loss after 30 months of follow-up (Surgery 98:700-707, 1985). In another study, 69% had fair-to-poor results in maintaining weight loss after 23 months and 22% suffered from obstruction of the narrow outlet from the stomach pouch (Mayo Clinic Proceedings 61:287-291, 1986). Weight regain after gastroplasty is usually the result of gradual stretching and enlargement of the stomach pouch or the narrow outlet from it. Because the stomach is almost infinitely expandable and adapts to increased pressure by growing larger, the operation is doomed to be eventually undone by natural adaptive processes of the patients' body. Although gastric bypass is more effective in maintaining loss of weight, there are more long-term complications, particularly nutritional deficiencies including anemia, pernicious anemia, osteoporosis, and neurological damage. These same complications were described 30 years ago as the long-term result of stomach surgery for ulcers. Consequently, these operations were long ago abandoned for treatment of ulcer.

The stomach is not simply a passive sac for storing ingested food, but plays a complex role in the processing of nutrients. Surgical procedures which interfere with the normal operation of the stomach inevitably cause multiple problems. Unfortunately, no controlled trials have ever been run which include physical examination of the patients for possible side effects by independent doctors not associated with the surgeon. In a rare instance of independent examination of bariatric surgery patient, a team of neurologists examined 500 patients who had received either gastric bypass or gastroplasty and found neurological complications (nerve or brain damage) in 5% of them (Neurology 37:196-200, 1987). The patients were usually examined within a year after surgery, so the incidence of long-term neurological deterioration could be much higher than 5%. Possible damage to organs other than brain and nervous system has not been put under rigorous independent evaluation.

Once a surgical technique has been developed in the animal laboratory, normally the next step is to run controlled clinical trials comparing long-term outcomes for patients and an untreated control group. Coronary bypass was tested in this way and it was proven that heart patients undergoing surgery lived longer than comparable patients getting only non-surgical treatment. No controlled clinical trials have ever been run for weight loss surgery, except for one Danish trial of gastric bypass that showed that patients undergoing surgery experienced more health problems than comparable patients who were put on very-low-calorie diets (New England Journal of Medicine 310:352-356, 1984; Danish Medical Bulletin 37:359-370, 1990). Gastric bypass or gastroplasty does result in improved levels of blood pressure, cholesterol, and blood sugar. These reduced risk factors might translate into long-term disease prevention over the patients' lifespan if (and only if) their reduced weight can be maintained for life.

Do the benefits of weight loss exceed the risks of major surgery and the side-effects of tampering with the digestive system? In considering this question, the consensus panel must first ask whether weight loss is permanent. If a patient loses 100 pounds only to gain it back five years later, then her risk factors will return to dangerous levels. Because of the harmful effects of losing and regaining weight (the "yo-yo syndrome"), some risk factors, especially blood pressure, may be worse after regain of weight than they were at the start. When the risks of surgery and long-term complications are taken into account, then it become apparent that the net outcome for the patient who regains weight is highly negative. The typical patient receiving these operations is a woman in her 30's. To be certain of reducing her risk for heart disease later in life, weight loss must be assured for at least 10 years and preferably 20.

The consensus panel must also consider the benefit side of the risk-benefit equation. In order to evaluate the benefits of weight loss in extremely obese persons, let us start with the

assumption that the poor health suffered by fat
people can be completely reversed by weight
loss. This may not be a valid assumption,
especially because it is now clear that many fat
people are burdened by a genetic defect that
allows runaway weight gain. This same genetic
defect may also lead to diabetes, high blood
pressure and heart disease. Currently we do not
know whether the health problems of the obese
are dire ctly caused by the fatty deposits
themselves or whether they result from defective
genetic machinery. If the latter is true, then weight
loss will not completely erase the excess risk
associated with obesity, because weight loss will
not change a person's genetic makeup. Setting
this argument aside, let us consider the actual risk
faced by extremely obese persons. The median
life expectancy from age 25 as a function of body
mass index is shown in the illustration above (see
original article). These data were taken from the
world's largest epidemiological study, which
tracked 1.8 million Norwegians for 10 years (Acta
Medica Scandinavica Supplementum 679:1-56,
1984). Let us consider the lifespan of women,
since 90-95% of all patients undergoing weight
loss surgery are female. Women who are neither
underweight nor overweight have a life
expectancy of about 79 years. Morbid obesity
begins at a body mass index of 35. Women with a
body mass index of 40 and above are shown at
the far right. Their life expectancy is reduced by 5
years, which is equivalent in risk to light cigarette
smoking. However, even these extremely obese
women still have a longer life expectancy that
normal-weight men. Several conclusions can be

made from this graph: first, the typical "morbidly obese" woman in her 30's considering weight loss surgery faces another four decades of life, which means that weight loss maintenance and surgical complications must be evaluated over the very long term. Second, given that the maximum benefit from weight loss is a 5-year prolongation of life, the risks from surgery must be kept very low. Third, surgery should clearly be reserved for the most obese patients (body mass index over 40) and the ongoing trend for surgeons to make exceptions to the "100-pound rule" and operate on thinner patients must be deplored.

The challenge awaiting the NIH consensus panel is formidable. They will lack a base of knowledge of the biological effects and the medical consequences of these operations, especially over the long term. The vast array of variations of these operations complicates any evaluation. Operations that are more effective are also less safe; none of the surgical procedures seem to be both safe and effective. Risks and benefits must be compared over the remaining 40 years of life expectancy of the patient, but for many procedures patients are tracked for two years or less, and many times only weight loss is recorded without independent evaluations of the patients' overall health. Hopefully the 1991 panel will not repeat the mistakes of the 1978 panel, which failed to confront the epidemic of complications from intestinal bypass.

Paul Ernsberger, Ph.D.
Associate Professor of Medicine, Pharmacology and Neuroscience Case Western Reserve School

of Medicine, 10900 Euclid Ave.,
Cleveland, OH 44106-4906
http://www.cwru.edu/med/nutrition/ernsberger.htm

A Nurses Perspective

I have given the nurse who wrote this article the name Sunshine because she offers a ray of hope to each of her patients. She is a highly qualified nurse and respected among her colleagues. I asked Sunshine to include her comments in my book so people can read a first hand account from a professional who has taken care of many patients with the gastric bypass surgery, including myself.

I am a registered nurse and have been one for four years. I have had the opportunity to care for many patients that have had the gastric bypass. In fact, I was the author's nurse when she had her bypass and I can tell you that her experiences are not unique. I have seen many patients that have had similar complications and far worse ones that those of the author.

When an overweight person approaches a doctor regarding the possibility of having a gastric bypass for the purpose of weight loss, there is a qualification process. The process differs from doctor to doctor, and for some doctors, the process is very simple. Doctors that are extremely thorough will have their patients consult with a nutritionist, psychologists, and other medical doctors to ensure that there is no other reason or treatment for the patient's obesity. Dr No, typically does not utilize these resources recommended by others. This particular doctor's qualification process is based on weight and the patient's desire to have the procedure done.

Many years ago, one of the qualifying factors for a gastric bypass of a stomach stapling was a weight that was at least 100 pounds over ideal body weight. Generally, Dr. No uses body mass index to qualify potential patients for the procedure. Body mass index (BMI) uses the patient's height and weight to determine a number that indicates the risk of health problems directly related to obesity. I am aware of patients of Dr. No's who had a BMI of 25 or greater. A BMI of 25 or lower indicates a low risk of health problems directly related to obesity. To put BMI into prospective, a person who is five feet tall and weighs 150 pounds has a BMI of about 30. According to Dr. No's criteria, this person would qualify for a gastric bypass. I will tell you that I have never cared for a patient with those statistics. The lightest patient that I have cared for was five feet three inches tall and weighed 220 pounds.

Another criterion for qualifying for a gastric bypass is having tried other weight loss programs. Most Americans, at some point in their lives, have been on some form of weight loss program. There are literally thousands of diet programs out there including Weight Watchers®, Overeaters Anonymous®, Optifast®, Slimfast®, and the Atkin's Diet® to name a few. Most doctors' want for their patients to have tried other forms of weight loss before they are qualified for surgery. The problem with this criterion is that there is really no way to prove how long a patient has tried these programs or how effective they truly are. Without a true analysis of a patient's diet by a nutritionist, determining a weight loss program that might be effective for the patient is impossible.

Part of my job as a nurse is to read the history and physical that is prepared by the doctor and is found on the patient's chart. Reading the history and physical helps me care for the patient by alerting me to coexisting conditions. Being aware of these conditions assists me in caring for my patients. For example, if I know that a patient is diabetic, I am alert to the possibility that the patient may at some point exhibit signs and symptoms of a high or low blood sugar.

The history and physical is a legal document and must be accurate. In my relationship with the author and in discussions with other patients, I have learned that the history and physicals of the doctor I am most familiar with were not always accurate. The author's history and physical said that she had two conditions that she had not experienced. Those conditions were high blood pressure and a rash under her abdominal fold.

Without exception, all of the history and physical reports that I read from this doctor included a histories of depression, joint problems, and a rash under the abdominal fold. All of these diagnoses were directly related to obesity. I will grant you that obesity can contribute to all of these conditions, but not everyone who is obese has them. In fact people who are not obese can and do have the same conditions.

I am now going to take some time to explain exactly what a gastric bypass is so that the reader may better understand the complications inherent in the procedure. Years ago, the weight loss surgery that was performed the most was a stomach stapling. In a stomach stapling, part of the stomach is removed and the remaining portion of the stomach is stapled back together. This creates a pouch that is smaller than the original stomach. The stomach is an organ that can be stretched and because of this, many people who had this procedure eventually stretched their stomachs back to originally size.

In a gastric bypass, the stomach is actually bypassed. A connection is made from the esophagus to the small intestine. Food does not enter the stomach after a gastric bypass; it goes directly into the small intestine. The small intestine does not stretch like the stomach does. Therefore, the pouch that is created does not enlarge like the stomach can. The pouch that is created generally holds between two and four ounces of food and/or fluid.

The stomach is an important organ for the digestion of protein. The stomach secretes and enzyme called pepsin that assists in protein digestion. If the stomach is bypassed, protein digestion becomes much more difficult.

As I mentioned earlier, the complications that the author experienced are not unique. During her stay in the hospital, the author progressed from surgery to discharge without complication. Immediate post-operative complications such as bleeding, infection, pneumonia, and leakage of intestinal fluid into the abdominal cavity are rare. I have seen all of these complications happen, but most patients survive the surgery without these problems. I have had the misfortune of seeing patients spend months in the hospital fighting to survive post-surgical complications, and have even watched some die.

Most of the complications that the author experienced are directly related to an altered gastrointestinal (GI) tract. Gastric bypass alters the GI tract and induces surgical starvation. We all know the dangers of starvation. We have all heard the stories about anorexics and may even know someone who is anorexic. Because gastric bypass is doctor supervised, we assume that it is safe and deny that it is starvation. The alteration of the GI tract that is induced by gastric bypass is permanent. It reduces the amount of space that a person has to absorb nutrients from the food that they eat. Even if the procedure is reversed, as in the author's case, the GI tract is still permanently altered. In this case, humpty-dumpty cannot be put back together.

Everyone who has a gastric bypass will suffer complications. Decreasing the amount of nutrients that we are able to absorb from the food that we eat will have adverse effects. Mild complications include food intolerances (particularly protein), hair loss (from protein malnutrition), nausea and vomiting, and activity intolerance. The more serious complications include muscle wasting, fluid and electrolyte imbalances, organ failure and death.

You have probably figured out by now that I am against gastric bypass. My feelings come not only from what I have seen in the clinical setting, but from what I have seen people in my personal life go through. I know several people who have had gastric procedures. In some cases these people initially did loss huge amounts of weight. In some cases though, they gained the weight back and then some. The weight loss induced is not always permanent. This occurs from the inability, or at least the reduced ability to digest protein. One of the easiest things for the body to digest is carbohydrates (starches and sugars). Anyone who is diabetic will tell you that they have to limit the amount of carbohydrate that they eat or they will gain weight. If all you are able to eat and keep down is carbohydrate, I guarantee that you will gain weight.

Losing weight can help alleviate or ease many health problems. However, surgical starvation trades old problems for new ones. There are other more healthful ways to lose weight.

The last thing that I will say is that if you are considering having a gastric bypass done, be sure that you are willing to accept the complications that I have mentioned here, including death. Are you willing to die weight?

23

Life Expectancy

If I knew then, what I know now, there is no way I would have had the gastric bypass surgery. The problems I had gone through during the eighteen months seemed insurmountable.

There is no scientific evidence the gastric bypass will give you a longer life.

When asking about how long will you live after WLS, the common answer for the lack of either long term patients or studies on longevity, is that the older WLS procedures are not done any more and the newer procedures are too new to determine.

This is somewhat misrepresentative. The most common procedure being done today is the RNY gastric bypass and it's not a new procedure, it was invented in the 1960's.

So where are all the post-ops today and where is the long term data on lifespan?

The gastric bypass has been done for 40 years and yet we have no long term data; no one seems to know any long term post ops, troubling to say the least.

On Lifespan after surgery:

1. Most deaths from gastric bypass are recorded as from other causes, including liver failure, aneurism, heart attack, and obesity. Very few deaths directly linkable to the gastric bypass are recorded as from the gastric bypass. Medical providers have said that this is not due to conspiracy, but because of the way the Medical Examiners' office works.

2. Livingston of UCLA Bariatric Center reported that multiple studies on patients, some over 8 years, had shown up to a 40 percent serious complication rate on the gastric bypass.

3. The Hebrew University study (1999 Israel), also a period of 8 years, showed that 70 percent of patients kept some weight off and 25 percent of patients gained back to near original weight and only about 7 percent of patients kept all excess weight off. This study did not report a number of deaths or complications.

4. The Mayo Clinic study, over 5 years, of proximal gastric bypass, showed a 20 percent rate of life threatening complications. It did not report death rate but stated that a significant number of patients 'fell off the study' each year (it was a survey study where patients were sent a survey at intervals and asked to fill out and send back). It is unknown what happened to those who failed to answer their survey.

5. The average lifespan after a Billroth II which the Alvarado clinic calls "physiologically similar" to the gastric bypass was 15-25 years.

WLS surgeons have given some statistics also. Probably the most accurate per se is that of Dr Walter Pories, MD in the Sabiston book on surgery which is used in medical schools. He reported that "now gastric bypass can be done with as low as a 1 death per 100 surgeries death rate". (1994) Dr Louis Flancbaum agrees with this statistic in his book, DOCTOR'S GUIDE TO Weight Loss Surgery (NY, 2001).

Sue Widemark states, "I have personally met 2 patients of gastric bypass surgery over 20 years. One is a BPD who has not revealed much about her state of health except to say she does have a very restrictive diet (no sweets, no carbs, etc) to keep her weight down. The other is a gastric bypass patient, 21 years out from surgery - who has colon cancer and just found out they also have 'massive bone mass loss'. They have alluded to other health issues as well. A JIB patient I've met (intestinal bypass) who is 26 years out from surgery is quite ill with autoimmune disease, multiple vitamin deficiencies etc. And another JIB, who was reversed in 1989, still has health issues and also says she knows several who died from the WLS. In fact, most of those who had surgery the same time as she did died".

It appears that since so many gastric bypass deaths are recorded as from other causes and since we know that some clinics are keeping detailed data over a several year period, but have not released the results. Is it possible the results of this data might show the surgery as less than what we are being told?

It is unknown why those results have not been released or what those results really are. Many people are coerced into a decision to have bariatric surgery by doctors who tell them they will be dead in 5 years if they don't have the surgery. Studies of 20,000 men by the Cooper Institute as well as studies of populations like the "PIMA Paradox" show us that *if a person exercises as little as 30 minutes, 3 times a week, their risk rate regardless of size, is way lower than a thin non-exerciser.*

But anyone who has obesity in their family has seen relatives who are large, live to a ripe old age. We've also seen WLS post ops die early. What is the answer to the longevity question? If those selling the surgery know, they probably will not tell US in the near future.

Doctor's have much more information then they are releasing to the public. A doctor has data on over 4,000 patients, but has not released it for public review. I wonder why we, who are seeking information, are not able to obtain everything that might help us make decisions regarding our lives. Why hide results unless they contain data that would stop the massive numbers of gastric bypass surgeries done in this country?

Before surgery, I was not told about how high the risks of further complications could be. Dr. No minimized my concerns when I brought up the subject and said, "I should not worry about that since any major problems seldom arose".

No one seems to be able to identify any long term patients (15 years out or more), not the surgeons and not the patients. Some clinics appear to be keeping data but to date have not released this information. Doctors should not be making claims they can't back up with accurate data.

Patients are asked to go to their weight loss surgeon for 3, 6, 9, and 12 month checkups during the first year following the gastric bypass surgery. After the first year, patients are told to go to their primary care physician for follow-up care and yearly blood tests. Many primary care physicians are left with taking care of their patients who can develop a host of problems. Many WLS surgeons seem concerned with only the weight loss. Dr Harvey Sugarman commented on this in the "Mayo Proceedings" Magazine – it is a source of concern to some. Although patients are told to return to their surgeons for 3, 6, 9 month checkups, often patients are either rushed through or not seen. In some cases, this has contributed to the death of a patient or left to those not familiar with this complex surgery, like a primary care physician. Sometimes, telling symptoms are not recognized in time to fix the problem. Yet all too often the primary care physicians and emergency room personnel are expected to pick up the pieces of patients lives.

24

Long Term Side

Affects

The side effects from the WLS had been much worse than Dr. No ever told me was possible. I have already listed several of these side affects that are not just an inconvenience, but life threatening. It isn't just an inconvenience to vomit daily; it can cause tearing of the esophagus, ripping of the staples lines, heart attacks, and more damage throughout the body.

According to the Pacific Institute of Surgery for Obesity (see Chapter 33 - References for URL), many long term side effects of the gastric bypass are unknown. They write (on their web site):

"The surgical treatment of obesity is an evolving process. We are learning and modifying techniques over time, resulting in more positive

*outcomes for our patients. Those complications
that have occurred provide us with new insights,
which are used to benefit future patients. Since
we don't yet have complete knowledge of long-
term results, we ask to see our patients in follow-
up for many years after the surgery."*

What is distressing is that many people don't
seem to fully explore the risks before ordering the
surgery, Wooley writes:

*"In today's climate it is naive to expect most
patients to show regard for their own health, so
over-riding is their desire for weight loss. This
issue has become particularly clear in the
experience gained with weight loss surgeries.
Many surgical candidates show a striking lack of
interest in the risks. After surgery, they ignore
severe and unpleasant side effects rather than
allow the procedure to be undone. 'Our female
patients', write Ravitch and Brolin (1979, pp 382-
391)' 'have been reluctant to accept the
dismantling procedure, even when it was
discussed in terms of SAVING THEIR LIVES.'"*

Patients with the WLS have reported they would
take any risk and ignore warnings of potential
problems in order to be thin. Some even have said
they would rather lose and arm or leg than to be fat.
Who knows why a person has such a low view of
themselves that they are willing to ignore life
threatening problems in order to wear a smaller size
of clothes. They traded one set of problems for
another and their lives are no better than before, and
too often -- much worse.

Will these people live as long as they have been told they would? I personally doubt it. There still isn't enough proof to verify people will live longer with the WLS. It seems obvious to me that eventually the body won't be able to take it any longer and give out. Those that profess to have no problems with their surgery haven't walked in the shoes of the very ill. The seriously ill don't see these long term problems as a little nuisance, instead, as a much lower quality of life. And, they were never told could happen.

While some regret having the WLS and the long term physical problems; others will always talk up the surgery as the best thing that ever happened to them, even if they are sick.

The long term health problems associated with the WLS are being reported as unrelated problems even though they are known symptoms. How can doctors report that patients will live longer and healthier lives with the WLS without clinical proof? If there is clinical data, it is not made available to the public. (The excuse usually made for the lack of long term clinical data is that the gastric bypass is a "new" surgery but the first gastric bypasses were done 40 years ago – this should have been enough time to amass a large body of long term data.)

The initial intent of the WLS was to help people who were morbidly obese become thinner and healthier. But, it turned out to be an experiment that went bad in my opinion. People who were desperate to be thin and healthy were and still are the guinea pigs in a weight loss industry that has been untruthful and secretive about the long term prognosis of these surgeries.

25

General Information

Not every overweight person is unhealthy and unable to have a happy life. I have seen overweight people more active than some thin people. Just because you are thin doesn't make you fit. However, some people do have severe health problems that this surgery could benefit.

I am concerned that the gastric bypass is being done far too often and on people that do not qualify. There are doctors who require patients to be at least 100 hundred pounds over their ideal weight before qualifying for the gastric bypass surgery. Then there are other doctors who will do the surgery on those that are 75 pounds over weight and less. It is not uncommon for people to purposely gain to meet the 100 pound mark in order to get the insurance company to approve the surgery.

A woman I know was refused by her insurance company three times because she didn't qualify for the weight loss surgery. Despite knowing of the risks with the surgery she wanted it anyway and was willing to do anything she could to get it. She even gained more weight, and ended up with diabetes, just to get insurance approval for her gastric bypass surgery. Her sister told her of a friend who died from the surgery, but that didn't sway her either. She was eventually approved by the insurance company and had the surgery. In my opinion, she should never have had this surgery based on her mental stability. According to this woman, she was encouraged to gain more weight and to put down on her medical history forms that she tried other methods of weight loss, when in fact she had not.

It is not hard for anyone to lie on their medical history forms filled out for their doctor if they want to have the gastric bypass surgery or any other WLS. Proof of these other methods that the potential WLS candidate has tried to lose weight can be easily verified via receipts of products bought or by programs they have enrolled in. I bring up this issue because I have known of people who are going to their primary care physicians asking for a referral for a quick way to get off weight. Dr. Caring told me numerous people are coming in and wanting the surgery without even trying any other method of controlling their weight.

I interviewed a woman who said, "I was told I wouldn't have to diet or exercise again with the RNY and I just don't want to change the way I eat and diet again. If the food isn't absorbed, I can eat, the calories will go right through me, and I will lose weight". What she failed to understand about the lack of absorbing is the danger it does to the body. If the food is passing through quickly, so are the nutrients from the food you need to sustaining life.

Patients with WLS are taking the supplements advised by their physician, but that is not good enough. They feel if they take all the recommended supplements they will be just fine and don't have to worry about long term deficiencies.

I was taking up to four times the recommended amounts of supplements and my naturopath still showed I wasn't getting enough when running rests on my system. His tests also showed I was not absorbing the calcium I needed to prevent osteoporosis. The tests he did on me indicated all my organs were under stress from the lack of absorption and malnutrition. There was no way to tell how long I could go without doing permanent damage to my organs. Instead of losing more weight, my body was drawing off nutrients from my organs. Even with the takedown of my gastric bypass I will always have to be monitored for long term damage to my body.

Losing more weight might make me look better, but it doesn't guarantee you will be healthier. Most people have a set point where their bodies stop losing, no matter how low they go in calories. This is often frustrating to people who either want to lose more weight or believe the doctor's charts. These charts are standards set by the medical community as to how much a person should weigh according to their height. I do not feel many doctors' take into account body type, genetics, and what weight a person can live at and still have a quality life.

The gastric bypass is a major surgery and every method of weight loss should be tried before altering the body. Even with the best doctor in the world you can still have complications. People's lives are not necessarily going to be better after having this surgery while others might. Some have a good experience while others end up an invalid or worse, they die.

People should also be thoroughly informed of possible physical and mental difficulties resulting from the gastric bypass surgery. Every person should have a psychological evaluation before the surgery. And, more than just a single hour visit, but several sessions to make sure all avenues have been explored. The WLS will not take care of emotional eating; it can make it worse. Even with a psychological exam there are still ways to get around the evaluation to get passed through. Some people I spoke with in the chat room who had the gastric bypass found the evaluations were so easy to get around. People can become quite convincing when they want something bad enough. Some will even be untruthful in order to pass the psychological evaluation to get the gastric bypass surgery. Dr. No didn't give a single psychological evaluation to his patients; feeling it was unnecessary. Dr. Compassion includes a psychological evaluation for all his patients.

A doctor and a qualified team should have available alternative treatments to chose from, and not just go to the gastric bypass surgery by default. If a patient has a medical problem that causes weight gain, then that needs to be addressed before even considering any type of invasive surgery. Weight gain can be due to depression, stress, anxiety, boredom, divorce, lack of self esteem, judgments from others, and so forth. None of these problems will go away with the WLS; they will still be there and need to be addressed. WLS surgery does not take care of emotional problems. Changing your shape won't necessarily change your life for the better.

The WLS surgery is not a cure-all for compulsive eating or any other eating disorder. If you can tolerate dairy products and eat cheese cake, a person can eat it several times a day and gain weight. The WLS can prevent you from eating large amounts of food, but not what you eat. This will be up to the person to make the changes in eating habits.

The WLS is a tool and I found that even using it properly, it still failed. I didn't have any eating disorders before the surgery, but found I had one afterwards. I did have to force myself to throw up if I got food stuck in the stoma, the pain was unbearable. The opening is only the size of a dime and is some cases, even smaller. Most of the time the vomiting was uncontrollable, this is called 'involuntary vomiting'. I never knew when anything I tried to eat would just fly out without warning. This is not normal and weakened my body every time I vomited. Whether I vomited to get food unstuck or had involuntary vomiting it still is under the classification of bulimia. The last thing I ever wanted is bulimia because of the damage it causes, and what I saw happen to two of my family members with this disorder.

The WLS does not address those with a genetic predisposition for weight gain. Before I had the gastric bypass surgery I could maintain my weight by eating 500 calories a day and after the surgery it was the same. I ate exactly what was recommend in order to be healthy and to lose weight, but still found it hard to maintain. On one hand, I wanted to eat and struggled with weight gain. On the other hand, it was easier to not eat because food was making me sick.

Even if people with the WLS eat correctly after having the gastric bypass surgery there still can be many problems that are unforeseen. Even the most qualified doctor with the best of intentions cannot guarantee the outcome for each patient.

Dr. Compassion is a professional I admire and trust. He didn't say he could guarantee my reversal would be perfect, but that he would do his best to help me get well. It was a risk I was willing to take after an extensive search into his qualifications. He is a man of integrity and has knowledge about the gastric bypass surgery and the reversal. After reviewing what he and his team put their patients through before doing the gastric bypass surgery, I now know I would never have qualified for the surgery.

I wish I had found Dr. Compassion when I was first looking into this surgery, but since that did not happen I can not go backwards and wonder what would have happened if I had. It was in the past and I was fortunate to find him to do my reversal.

After I had the gastric bypass surgery, and then the reversal, I had decided not to have any surgery done to remove excess skin. Going through any more surgeries was way too much for me to even think about. Besides, I was happy with the way I looked and never wanted to look like a Barbie Doll.

Those that have lost several hundred pounds often have a medical reason for the skin removal, such as rashes under the skin folds. I did want to find out more about the plastic surgery people have chosen to remove excess skin. I spoke with two Plastic Surgeons; I will call Nip and Tuck. They both conveyed to me they do not want to do any reconstruction on patients until they had kept off their weight for at least two years. Some doctors' do it sooner while others wait for more time to pass because of the dangers. If weight is regained there can be problems of stretching and ripping of the scar tissue around the incision as well as internal tearing.

If a woman is thinking of getting pregnant, both doctors stated they would not remove excess skin. Pregnancy can put a great deal of pressure on the incision so it is best to wait until a woman is through having children.

Nip said he will not do any skin removal on people who have had the gastric bypass surgery because the chance of regaining weight is so high. Tuck said he would do reconstructive surgery on patients with the gastric bypass surgery. But only when they have stabilized their weight loss, which he said would require at least two years or more.

Quick massive weight loss usually causes large amounts of loose skin (the body has not had time to adjust the skin to accommodate less body mass). Many WLS post ops start getting into the 'plastic surgery' syndrome. Usually a 'tummy tuck' is needed to rid the person of loose skin around the middle – many have loose skin and tucks elsewhere on the body and some even have liposuction and face lifts.

It should be remembered that all surgery has the potential of being dangerous. Some WLS post-ops get through the initial surgery alright, and then have a lot of trouble and/or pain with the 'tummy tuck' (drainage for several weeks is common – sometimes bleeding occurs).

While some doctors say weight loss from the gastric bypass is permanent, others are reporting some weight gain on the patients they keep in contact with. What about all the patients that are no longer going to their doctor after their one year check-up? In a study at Hebrew University on proximal gastric bypass, it was found that 24 percent of the patients gained back to very large size and only 7 percent of the patients were able to keep all their weight off.

There are doctors' reporting 90 percent of their patients are able to keep off the weight loss after fifteen years. If this is so, why are patients having their gastric bypass redone more than once? Some are having a second and a third surgery because they gained back the weight they lost. This surgery has been done on patients for over forty years, so I ask; where are the statistics on those patients? I have seen some data showing as low as 50 percent regain their weight and another place showing as much as 90 percent regain after five years. Surgeons consider a bariatric patient a success if they retain 40 percent of the initial weight loss. This means a person who weighs 370 pounds can lose 205 pounds, gain back 123 pounds, now weighing 288 pounds – and can be still counted as a 'success' by the bariatric surgeon. It's easy to see where they can conclude that 90 or more percent of gastric bypass patients are a "success" in keeping the weight off.

Several people I have spoken to have said they will not go back to their doctor who did their gastric bypass surgery because they gained their weight back and did not want to be considered a failure. One woman said she has had three gastric bypass surgeries because she kept gaining back the weight. Her doctor refused to do any more on her, a wise decision.

The woman who had all these gastric bypass surgeries felt the surgery would take care of all her problems and she would never have to diet again. Wrong! People go in with the expectation they will not have to diet again, but the reality is quite the opposite. If patients with the WLS have to diet and exercise to get the weight off and keep it off for the rest of their lives, why not do it without the surgery.

Talk on the on-line support groups lists often includes 'joining Weight Watchers', 'joining Overeaters anonymous', or 'taking diet pills'. In addition to having to do something they found annoying before surgery (dieting and exercising), WLS post-ops must, for the rest of their lives, deal with the daily problems from surgery such as dumping (a hypoglycemic reaction), food getting stuck in the stoma, malnutrition, mal-absorption, organ failure, regaining weight, eating disorders, and much more.

This surgery is one that will change your life and it's very important to do extensive research before making this decision. Even when you do think you have done all your homework and have all the information available, it might not be enough to make an informed decision. If there is any doubt, don't do it.

26

Eating Disorders

The following is information about eating disorders and treatment by The National Institute of Mental Health. It is important to gain knowledge about these disorders before making a decision about having WLS because this surgery will not take care of these problems and could make them worse.

Many people want to have the WLS to change the outside of them while not addressing what is going on in the inside. Getting help for an eating disorder may solve the problem without the surgery. The RNY produces an involuntary form of bulimia. Vomiting from nausea, food being stuck in the stoma, drinking liquids with solid food, and vomiting to lose weight and keep it off.

I have spoken with several patients of the RNY who worry about regaining weight and vomit to keep their weight off. They disregard the medical problems associated with the chronic vomiting, and continue to eat and purge.

Eating is controlled by many factors, including appetite, food availability, family, peers, and cultural practices, and attempts at voluntary control. Dieting to a body weight leaner than needed for health is highly promoted by current fashion trends, sales campaigns for special foods, and in some activities and professions.

Eating disorders involve serious disturbances in eating behavior, such as extreme and unhealthy reduction of food intake or severe overeating, as well as feelings of distress or extreme concern about body shape or weight. Researchers are investigating how and why initially voluntary behaviors, such as eating smaller or larger amounts of food than usual, at some point move beyond control in some people and develop into an eating disorder.

Studies on the basic biology of appetite control and its alteration by prolonged overeating or starvation have uncovered enormous complexity, but in the long run have the potential to lead to new pharmacologic treatments for eating disorders.

Eating disorders are not due to a failure of will or behavior; rather, they are real, treatable medical illnesses in which certain maladaptive patterns of eating take on a life of their own. The main types of eating disorders are anorexia nervosa and bulimia nervosa. A third type, binge-eating disorder, has been suggested, but has not yet been approved as a formal psychiatric diagnosis. Eating disorders frequently develop during adolescence or early adulthood, but some reports indicate their onset can occur during childhood or later in adulthood.

Eating disorders frequently co-occur with other psychiatric disorders such as depression, substance abuse, and anxiety disorders. In addition, people who suffer from eating disorders can experience a wide range of physical health complications, including serious heart conditions and kidney failure which may lead to death. Recognition of eating disorders as real and treatable diseases, therefore, is critically important.

Females are much more likely than males to develop an eating disorder. Only an estimated 5 to 15 percent of people with anorexia or bulimia and an estimated 35 percent of those with binge-eating disorder are male.

Anorexia Nervosa

An estimated 0.5 to 3.7 percent of females suffer from anorexia nervosa in their lifetime. Symptoms of anorexia nervosa include:

- Resistance to maintaining body weight at or above a minimally normal weight for age and height.

- Intense fear of gaining weight or becoming fat, even though underweight.

- Disturbance in the way in which one's body weight or shape is experienced, undue influence of body weight or shape on self-evaluation, or denial of the seriousness of the current low body weight.

- Infrequent or absent menstrual periods (in females who have reached puberty).

People with this disorder see themselves as overweight even though they are dangerously thin. The process of eating becomes an obsession. Unusual eating habits develop, such as avoiding food and meals, picking out a few foods and eating these in small quantities, or carefully weighing and portioning food. People with anorexia may repeatedly check their body weight, and many engage in other techniques to control their weight, such as intense and compulsive exercise, or purging by means of vomiting and abuse of laxatives, enemas, and diuretics. Girls with anorexia often experience a delayed onset of their first menstrual period.

The course and outcome of anorexia nervosa varies across individuals: Some fully recover after a single episode; some have a fluctuating pattern of weight gain and relapse; and, others experience a chronically deteriorating course of illness over many years. The mortality rate among people with anorexia has been estimated at 0.56 percent per year, or approximately 5.6 percent per decade, which is about 12 times higher than the annual death rate due to all causes of death among females ages 15-24 in the general population. The most common causes of death are complications of the disorder, such as cardiac arrest, electrolyte imbalance, or suicide.

Bulimia Nervosa

An estimated 1.1 percent to 4.2 percent of females have bulimia nervosa in their lifetime. Symptoms of bulimia nervosa include:

- Recurrent episodes of binge eating, characterized by eating an excessive amount of food within a discrete period of time and by a sense of lack of control over eating during the episode.

- Recurrent inappropriate compensatory behavior in order to prevent weight gain, such as self-induced vomiting or misuse of laxatives, diuretics, enemas, or other medications (purging); fasting; or excessive exercise.

- The binge eating and inappropriate compensatory behaviors both occur, on average, at least twice a week for 3 months.

- Self-evaluation is unduly influenced by body shape and weight.

Because purging or other compensatory behavior follows the binge-eating episodes, people with bulimia usually weigh within the normal range for their age and height. However, like individuals with anorexia, they may fear gaining weight, desire to lose weight, and feel intensely dissatisfied with their bodies. People with bulimia often perform the behaviors in secret, feeling disgusted and ashamed when they binge, yet relieved once they purge.

Binge-Eating Disorder

Community surveys have estimated that between 2 percent and 5 percent of Americans experience binge-eating disorder in a 6-month period. Symptoms of binge-eating disorder include:

- Recurrent episodes of binge eating, characterized by eating an excessive amount of food within a discrete period of time and by a sense of lack of control over eating during the episode.

- The binge-eating episodes are associated with at least 3 of the following; eating much more rapidly than normal; eating until feeling uncomfortably full; eating large amounts of food when not feeling physically hungry; eating alone because of being embarrassed by how much one is eating; feeling disgusted with oneself, depressed, or very guilty after overeating.

- Marked distress about the binge-eating behavior.

- The binge eating occurs, on average, at least 2 days a week for 6 months.

- The binge eating is not associated with the regular use of inappropriate compensatory behaviors (e.g., purging, fasting, excessive exercise).

People with binge-eating disorder experience frequent episodes of out-of-control eating, with the same binge-eating symptoms as those with bulimia. The main difference is that individuals with binge-eating disorder do not purge their bodies of excess calories. Therefore, many with the disorder are overweight for their age and height. Feelings of self-disgust and shame associated with this illness can lead to bingeing again, creating a cycle of binge eating.

Treatment Strategies

Eating disorders can be treated and a healthy weight restored. The sooner these disorders are diagnosed and treated, the better the outcomes are likely to be. Because of their complexity, eating disorders require a comprehend-sive treatment plan involving medical care and monitoring, psychosocial interventions, nutritional counseling and, when appropriate, medication management. At the time of diagnosis, the clinician must determine whether the person is in immediate danger and requires hospitalization.

Treatment of anorexia calls for a specific program that involves three main phases; (1) restoring weight lost to severe dieting and purging; (2) treating psychological disturbances such as distortion of body image, low self-esteem, and interpersonal conflicts; and (3) achieving long-term remission and rehabilitation, or full recovery. Early diagnosis and treatment increases the treatment success rate. Use of psychotropic medication in people with anorexia should be considered *only* after weight gain has been established. Certain selective serotonin reuptake inhibitors (SSRIs) have been shown to be helpful for weight maintenance and for resolving mood and anxiety symptoms associated with anorexia.

The acute management of severe weight loss is usually provided in an inpatient hospital setting, where feeding plans address the person's medical and nutritional needs. In some cases, intravenous feeding is recommended. Once malnutrition has been corrected and weight gain has begun, psychotherapy (often cognitive-behavioral or interpersonal psychotherapy) can help people with anorexia overcome low self-esteem and address distorted thought and behavior patterns. Families are sometimes included in the therapeutic process.

The primary goal of treatment for bulimia is to reduce or eliminate binge eating and purging behavior. To this end, nutritional rehabilitation, psychosocial intervention, and medication management strategies are often employed. Establishment of a pattern of regular, non-binge meals, improvement of attitudes related to the eating disorder, encouragement of healthy but not excessive exercise, and resolution of co-occurring conditions such as mood or anxiety disorders are among the specific aims of these strategies. Individual psychotherapy (especially cognitive-behavioral or interpersonal psychotherapy), group psychotherapy that uses a cognitive-behavioral approach, and family or marital therapy have been reported to be effective. Psychotropic medications, primarily antidepressants such as the selective serotonin reuptake inhibitors (SSRIs), have been found helpful for people with bulimia, particularly those with significant symptoms of depression or anxiety, or those who have not responded adequately to psychosocial treatment alone. These medications also may help prevent relapse. The treatment goals and strategies for binge-eating disorder are similar to those for bulimia, and studies are currently evaluating the effectiveness of various interventions.

People with eating disorders often do not recognize or admit that they are ill. As a result, they may strongly resist getting and staying in treatment. Family members or other trusted individuals can be helpful in ensuring that the person with an eating disorder receives needed care and rehabilitation. For some people, treatment may be long term.

Research Findings and Directions

Research is contributing to advances in the understanding and treatment of eating disorders.

- NIMH-funded scientists and others continue to investigate the effectiveness of psychosocial interventions, medications, and the combination of these treatments with the goal of improving outcomes for people with eating disorders.

- Research on interrupting the binge-eating cycle has shown that once a structured pattern of eating is established, the person experiences less hunger, less deprivation, and a reduction in negative feelings about food and eating. The two factors that increase the likelihood of bingeing—hunger and negative feelings—are reduced, which decreases the frequency of binges.

- Several family and twin studies are suggestive of a high heritability of anorexia and bulimia, and researchers are searching for genes that confer susceptibility to these disorders. Scientists suspect that multiple genes may interact with environmental and other factors to increase the risk of developing these illnesses. Identification of susceptibility genes will permit the development of improved treatments for eating disorders.

- Other studies are investigating the neurobiology of emotional and social behavior relevant to eating disorders and the neuroscience of feeding behavior.

- Scientists have learned that both appetite and energy expenditure are regulated by a highly complex network of nerve cells and molecular messengers called neuropeptides. These and future discoveries will provide potential targets for the development of new pharmacologic treatments for eating disorders.

- Further insight is likely to come from studying the role of gonadal steroids. Their relevance to eating disorders is suggested by the clear gender effect in the risk for these disorders, their emergence at puberty or soon after, and the increased risk for eating disorders among girls with early onset of menstruation.

27

What's Next?

Many diets have been tried and billions of dollars have been spent over the years on weight loss programs and products. Very few, if any, have proved successful except to empty our wallets and dash our hopes of succeeding at losing weight.

There have been numerous pills, over the counter and ones dispensed by physicians. Patients initially would lose weight, only to regain it all, and then some. Many of the pills caused long term health problems, including heart disease as the predominate ailment. Death occurred in many people who were just trying to get excess weight off and use these magical pills to take care of the problem.

There was a time people wired their mouths shut and took in only liquids until the weight came off. They soon found out after the wires were off and could eat food again, and the weight came right back on. This procedure was considered safe and with a long term success rate, but this turned out to be false.

There are liquid proteins and other drinks that are thought to be a quick way to loose weight, but they haven't had long lasting success.

There have been all the fad diets that failed to help people lose weight and keep it off. The grapefruit diet, banana diet, cabbage diet, hot dog diet, and many more too numerous to even mention. There are programs that provide pre-packaged food at a high cost and counting points for food. Everywhere we look; there is another weight loss program to try. No one can blame people from trying to gain control over their weight issues. Each diet tried and failed leaves a person feeling more of a failure, hope is dashed once again. No one is a failure for trying a diet, they aren't meant to be long lasting, they line the pockets of business that's sole purpose is to make money at all costs.

Corporate money isn't being spent on those who can't get to a gym or are incapacitated. The government picks up the tab when all else fails, so we all pay. Companies are making money by promoting their cure-all for weight problems, even when they don't work. They feed on people's guilt, fears, and threat of dying if the weight isn't taken off. I encourage a balanced way of eating and probably the most important aspect is including exercise.

I tend to get bored easily if I do only one form of exercise so I include a variety of programs. One day I might hike in the mountains, the next day go to gym and ride a stationary bike or swim laps. I also include Yoga and Tai Chi for my physical and mental Well being. Along with my exercising, which kicks in the endorphins and increases the metabolism, I eat what I want and will not ever diet again. I continue to eat very small portions and a low calorie count because my body just doesn't need much food. I do avoid high calorie foods because energy in needs to be translated to energy out. I think very carefully before taking a bite of a cookie or something else that is high calorie since I know how far I have to walk to wear it off. I also look at why I eat, or feel a need for the food and not what I eat. The way I take care of myself isn't a diet, it is a way of life and I don't see it as a punishment.

Diets don't work! They only set people up for failure and you can't diet for life. Diets are temporary and often throw us into the yo-yo syndrome. Down in weight, up in weight, and the cycle continues which is unhealthier than if you didn't lose and regain on a continuous basis. Each time a diet is tried the metabolism is affected. Low calorie intake slows the metabolism so weight gain is even easier than before a diet. The body says, hey I am being starved, so I better hang on to the weight I've got.

The first three letters of diet are DIE and that is what happens to our spirits every time we try another method of weight loss and it doesn't work.

In my mind, the WLS is a diet, it is meant to prohibit the absorption of food. It restricts the amount of food taken in and will not work without exercise and constant monitoring of calories. Who wouldn't lose weight on 300 calories a day and with an hour or two of exercising. As I see it, the major issue with the WLS is health problems and they are insurmountable.

When people talk about what has gone wrong with them since having the WLS it doesn't seem like the problems are minor in many cases.

I haven't seen any proof that the first, second, and third, versions of the weight loss surgery were deemed safe and healthy. All were proclaimed safe and healthy, but all have had major downsides to the procedures. Is the WLS just another fad diet that will eventually go the way all the rest have gone? It won't go away as long as money is to be made and people are willing to put themselves through these surgeries.

The adjustable lap band now being performed on patients is a less invasive procedure and has the same weight loss as some of the others. This procedure still does not guarantee you will keep the weight off. It takes a change in life style when approaching long term results in weight loss and maintenance. However, the advantage of the adjustable lap band (AGB) is that it is FULLY reversible, and there is no stomach stapling or intestinal re-routing included. A disadvantage would be that the adjustable band can interfere with the Lower Espohagal Spinctor (LES) from opening and thus interfere with the perestalsis (muscle wave) in the esophagus. That means food can get stuck for a while and can be painful. This surgery is not without complications and there have been reported deaths.

There is a new procedure coming out called, Gastric Pacing, much like the heart pace maker, but located in the stomach. It will be done through laparoscopy and will send signals to the stomach, letting you know you are full with less food. This procedure is being tested now in Europe and will become available in the United States sometime in the year 2003 or 2004. Again, it still does involve anesthesia and small openings into the body. There is also a foreign object placed in the body and no way of know if it will be rejected.

Liposuction has been provided to patients as a means to reduce weight instantly for several years and is widely used today. There are serious side affects to this surgery, such as, loss of fluids, bleeding, and death. It is not to be taken lightly and done only by an experienced doctor.

Again, do your research into the procedure and make sure the physician is board certified. Ask for a list of former and current patients to talk with. Family doctors can also help refer you to a competent specialist.

One of the most horrific weight loss procedures being made available is the administering of 'Pharmaceutical Tape Worms' into a patient. Once the worms are placed into the patient they will eat up the food being consumed. When the patient has lost the desired weight, the worms are destroyed through medication, and then they pass out of the body. There is weight loss from this method, but in my opinion, the thought of having worms inside me wiggling around is enough to make me not want to ever eat again.

But then again, many have resorted to having the gastric bypass surgery that alters the stomach and digestive tract to help lose weight. The worms are temporary and the WLS is not always reversible, depending on which surgery has been performed.

Diets can work for the short term. But, what is important is the long run. Food can be used for comfort in times of stress; it can be used to fill an empty void within, or used to put on weight for protection. Looking at the reasons why one eats the amount or kinds of food is important before asking the body to change an old pattern for a new one that is healthier. A change in life style is still the best way to lose weight and keep it off for life. I hear people every day say they have tried every diet and they all failed so want the weight loss surgery. Believe me, after you have been sliced and diced and end up with several complications you will look at the old fashion way of losing weight as much easier.

Food is not the enemy; it is nourishment that feeds our bodies. Not all weight loss programs are failures. Some have long term success rates, but they depend on the person being able to stick with it for life.

The following is a comparison between a "low fat with a daily exercise program" and the "weight loss surgery" after three years. Both may work, but the non-surgical solution is healthier if you are able to do it.

Low Fat Diet with Daily Exercise	Weight Loss Surgery (WLS)
You will have lost 100 to 150 lbs.	You will have lost 100 to 150 lbs.
You will have to exercise daily to keep your weight off.	You will have to exercise daily to keep your weight off.
You will be very strong and healthy with lots of energy.	You might have less energy due to inability to eat much food.
Your metabolism will be higher than it's ever been due to muscle forming and that means you can eat more without gaining your weight back.	Your metabolism may be lower than it's ever been due to chronic starvation and that means you might not be able to eat more than 800-1000 calories a day without gaining weight.
You will have no vitamin deficiencies.	You might have B12, calcium and other vitamin deficiencies which require regular injections and/or supplements.
You can get enough calcium if you drink 3 glasses of milk a day or the equivalent.	You may have difficulty absorbing calcium and are likely at risk for osteoporosis in your fifties or sixties (like most Americans).

Low Fat Diet with Daily Exercise	Weight Loss Surgery (WLS)
You will have enough iron in your blood.	You might have an iron deficiency.
You can easily get pregnant and give your baby all the nutrients s/he needs to be a healthy baby. You will be healthy also.	You can easily get pregnant, but might have problems supplying the baby (or yourself) with nutrients due to reduced ability to eat.
You will have to see your doctor about once a year for a checkup.	You will probably need to be regularly monitored by your physician.
You can enjoy a good meal and even cheat on holidays.	You may not be able to enjoy a full meal (this varies with the individual, but the fear of gaining is also a factor).
You can have a piece (even two) of your birthday cake.	You'd better skip the cake due to a danger of dumping - eat some green beans instead.

28

Things to Consider

The following is a list of things to consider before deciding if the weight loss surgery is for you or not. (provided by Sue Widemark)

1. A gastric bypass is not only a 'stomach stapling' as the media is fond of calling it. It's also an intestinal bypass. In a proximal bypass, only about 20 inches of small intestine is bypassed, but that includes the Duodenum in which most of the absorption of vitamins and minerals takes place. This means that even with a small amount of intestine bypassed, the post op might develop vitamin and mineral deficiencies.

2. Calcium deficiency: The only place the body can take in calcium is in the duodenum part of the small intestine - this is totally bypassed in all gastric bypasses except the 'duodenal switch' (in which 1-2 inches are left - probably not enough to do any more than absorb some sugar and prevent

calcium supplements you take, research has shown that your body might not be able to access it. And this means, you have a strong probability of coming down with osteoporosis sometime after the sixth year post op.

3. The newest studies show that gastric bypass patients lack a hormone called "Ghrelin" in their bloodstream. This hormone is known to encourage the production of "human growth hormone (HGH)". *The lack of this hormone (and consequently no HGH) in gastric bypass patients may explain the fact that most seem to age greatly after their gastric bypass.* HGH is considered the key factor in our aging process - the less we have, the more we age.

   You will have to supplement other vitamins like B12 and iron for the rest of your life. B12 is best taken in 'shots'. This is because your digestive system no longer digests or absorbs many vitamins and nutrients.

4. You might have to go back to the hospital for repeat surgeries for hernias, bowel obstruction (this is very painful until you have the surgery done) and scopes (tubes down your throat to see if all if ok). Some WLS post ops also have a lot of plastic surgery because the original surgery does not give them the svelte figure they imagined it would.

5. Gastric bypass patients don't have much appetite because it is difficult to eat and they often are nauseous. Think of eating food when the opening for the food to leave the pouch is very small. Everything has to be chewed very well. Because if

it gets stuck in the opening leading to the small gut, it can cause very intense pain until it dissolves. Occasionally patients have to go to the hospital to get the food removed surgically.

6. Bad gut bugs: After your stomach is made very small, it will not produce much acid anymore. This is done to save acid from burning your esophagus. The downside is that the bacteria in the food do not get killed and can get into the blood stream. This is called "leaky gut" and is suspected to cause autoimmune disorders like LUPUS, rheumatoid arthritis and even in rare cases, multiple sclerosis. Since you may have a lot of bacteria getting into your blood, you might be sick more often after weight loss surgery.

7. Restrictive diet and exercise: Some people go into surgery because they think the procedure will work automatically. The reality is that after the first year, gastric bypass patients will likely face dieting and exercise to maintain their new physique. The restrictive diet includes no fat, no sugar - much more restrictive than is necessary without surgery! (The "Hebrew University Study" showed that 25 % of those patients surveyed, gained back all their weight within 6 years. Only 7 % of those surveyed kept off ALL the weight that they lost)

Some post-ops who are four and five years out from surgery, do stay fairly thin, but only because they have a lot of physical problems. Be careful that you aren't exchanging one set of problems for another. Cancer will make you thin also, but that doesn't mean it's something a person would want to have.

8. Weight Loss Surgery will not fix depression. As a matter of fact, prolonged starvation (which you will experience, eating 500-1000 calories a day and not absorbing much in the way of nutrients) has been observed to cause depression.

9. The reason you start to gain weight after a year or so, is because your body has set your metabolism way down due to the prolonged starvation for the first year. Your body does this by cannibalizing its own muscles and even parts of organs. There is a growing body of evidence that starvation can cause brain damage and a lessening of mental abilities as well. This would make sense as the brain is not necessary to maintain life. (Some surgeons suggest doing tests to make sure your body is burning muscle and organ parts - instead of fat - so that you get the proper amount of protein in those months after surgery when you are not eating very much...- see the Scopinaro study on www.duodenalswitch.com)

10. According to what statistics are known (although the gastric bypass has been being done for over 40 years, not many long term post ops are to be found), about 1 out of every 200 who has the surgery, dies from complications. There is also some evidence that many deaths during the first year after surgery may be attributed to other causes like 'obesity'. This would possibly make the statistics incorrect, i.e., the death rate might be and probably is, much higher than those selling the surgery are willing to admit.

11. Success stories on websites are usually newly post op. All diets have their group of 'camp

followers' who are successful with the diet and say it's great. Weight Loss surgery (which IS a diet) is no different. But most of the camp followers are less than three years out from surgery.

Some rheumatologists seem to feel that the high prevalence of rheumatoid arthritis, joint disease and the like they see in post op WLS patients IS connected to the surgery. A rare complication also seen a few years after surgery is a partial paralysis, usually of the legs called "neuropathy". B12 deficiency can cause autoimmune disease like LUPUS.

12. Reversing the procedure: Today's surgeries are meant to be permanent. This is because in most of them, the stomach is partially destroyed. This is why surgeons talk about a "take down" rather than a reversal. A person requiring a takedown usually has a difficult time finding a surgeon to DO one. A person should realize that once they have had the surgery, even with a 'takedown' they will have repercussions for the rest of their lives.

13. Is Surgery the only way? Will you die without it? Numerous studies of obese people show that if they exercise and eat a reasonably healthy diet, they can remain large and still be healthy.

14. If you have a proximal gastric bypass, you will probably begin gaining weight after 12 to 18 months. For this reason, some patients have distal bypasses and BPD (bileopancreatic diversions). In this type of bypass, over 50 percent of the small intestine is bypassed, not that much different from the old (and dangerous) intestinal bypass! If you have this drastic surgery, there is a good chance

that you might develop severe nutritional deficiencies due to lack of absorption. Many surgeons will not do distal bypasses and BPDs for this reason. Although they've refined the operation somewhat by closing off the bypassed intestine, there are no guarantees of not having the nasty side effects seen in the older surgeries.

15. Liver failure: Patients are told that the old 'intestinal bypass' is no longer done due to the high incidence of liver failure in patients. However, many post op gastric bypass patients have elevated liver enzymes, a sign of liver damage. There are no guarantees that the gastric bypass won't also cause liver failure long term.

16. Stomach Cancer: According to medical books, anyone whose stomach is cut open, cut in two or surgically modified (called a 'gastrectomy') is of much higher risk for stomach cancer.

17. According to the ASBS website: "Any procedure involving mal-absorption must be considered at risk to develop at least some of the mal-absorptive complications exemplified by JIB (jejuno-ileal bypass)." All gastric bypasses work partially through mal-absorption so the following complications might (according to the ASBS) be seen with the modern gastric bypass:

Listing of jejuno-ileal bypass complications:

Mineral and Electrolyte Imbalance:

Decreased serum sodium, potassium, magnesium and bicarbonate.

Osteoporosis and osteomalacia secondary to protein depletion, calcium and vitamin D loss, and acidosis,

Protein Calorie Malnutrition:

Hair loss, anemia, edema, and vitamin depletion

Cholelithiasis:

Enteric Complications:

Abdominal distension, irregular diarrhea, increased flatus, pneumatosis intestinalis, colonic pseudo-obstruction, bypass enteropathy, volvulus with mechanical small bowel obstruction.

Extra-intestinal Manifestations:

Arthritis

Acute liver failure may occur in the postoperative period, and may lead to death acutely following surgery.

Liver disease, occurs in at least 30%

Steatosis, "alcoholic" type hepatitis, cirrhosis, occurs in 5%, progresses to cirrhosis and death in 1-2%

Erythema Nodosum, non-specific pustular dermatosis

Weber-Christian Syndrome

Renal Disease: (in other words, kidney disease and kidney failure)

Hyperoxaluria, with oxalate stones or interstitial oxalate deposits, immune complex nephritis, "functional" renal failure.

Miscellaneous:

Peripheral neuropathy, pericarditis, pleuritis, hemolytic anemia, neutropenia, and thrombocytopenia.

It should be noted that all surgeries are not equal. A new surgery, the Adjustable Band, has just been approved by the FDA. This is the most often done for weight loss surgery in Europe. Although there are no statistics on long term repercussions, this surgery, unlike the others is reversible. The stomach is not destroyed in any way. The band is not complication free by any means, and there is some evidence that it's rather uncomfortable to live with at times. However, the success rates with the adjustable band are similar to those seen with the gastric bypass.

As with all things, if in doubt, don't. You can always have the surgery at a later date when you have a greater comfort level about it.

The following is a list of contraindications for Weight loss surgery. It is a general guide to be reviewed with your surgeon. Check with your doctor about any one of these issues if you have a question.

Contraindications

Weight loss surgery may not be right for you if:

1. You have an inflammatory disease or condition of the gastrointestinal tract, such as ulcers, severe esophagitis, or Crohn's disease.

2. You have severe heart or lung disease that makes you a poor candidate for surgery.

3. You have some other disease that makes you a poor candidate for surgery, for example Addison's disease.

4. You have a problem that could cause bleeding in the esophagus or stomach. That might include esophageal or gastric varices (a dilated vein). It might also be something such as congenital or acquired intestinal telangiectasia (dilation of a small blood vessel).

5. You have portal hypertension.

6. Your esophagus, stomach, or intestine is not normal (congenital or acquired). For instance you might have a narrowed opening. .

7. You have cirrhosis (sick liver).

8. You have chronic pancreatitis.

9. You are pregnant. (If you become pregnant after the BioEnterics LAP-BAND System has been placed, the band may need to be deflated. The same is true if you need more nutrition for any other reason, such as becoming seriously ill. In rare cases, removal may be needed.) If you have a gastric bypass, the vitamins your body is not absorbing from food may be leeched from organs like the heart or the baby may suffer.

10. You are addicted to alcohol or drugs.

11. You are under 18 years of age or over 60 years of age.

12. You have an infection anywhere in your body or one that could contaminate the surgical area.

13. You are on chronic, long-term steroid treatment.

14. You cannot or do not want to follow the dietary rules that come with this procedure.

15. You or someone in your family has an autoimmune connective tissue disease. That might be a disease such as systemic lupus erythematosus or scleroderma, or multiple sclerosis. The same is true if you have symptoms of one of these diseases.

16. You have an eating disorder like bulimia.

29

Pre Op Questions

The following comments, concerns, and questions were communicated to me in person, telephone conversations, and through e-mails. The answers I give are my own and not from any medical institution or doctor.

1. Will the weight I lose with the WLS be permanent?

    According to the people I have spoken with, many doctors tell their patients the weight they lose is permanent. But this turns out to not be the case. When the 'honeymoon' period is over, which is different for each person, weight can come right back on. The 'honeymoon' period is the time you lose weight and this usually is within the first and second year of the surgery. I stopped losing after ten months; no matter how little I was able to get in. There is no guarantee you will keep off the weight and many seek revisions to the surgery so they can continue to lose weight or lose what they gained back. Many people with the WLS struggle to maintain weight loss after the surgery just like any other diet.

2. Will I ever have to diet and exercise again?

Yes, it will always be a part of your life and even more so after having any WLS. With months of malnutrition the body's metabolism is less effective than ever before. Many WLS patients go to Weight Watchers, take diet pills, and back to all the other programs they tried before they had the surgery.

Eating properly is more important after having any form of WLS because the body lacks the ability to absorb nutrients. Exercise is a must, but often difficult for patients who are too ill to participate in any activity. Without exercising a patient will have a higher rate of weight gain, with or without the surgery.

3. Will WLS help with eating disorders, like binging?

No, if you had an eating disorder before WLS you will still have it afterwards. This is one reason why people gain back their weight; they haven't dealt with an eating disorder before they had the surgery. To get in enough food most patients need to eat often. This can start a cycle of grazing, eating small amounts of food several times a day. If the stomach gets stretched, which it does in many cases, the weight comes back on with the increase in food. If a person has a problem with binging they will still have this problem after surgery. Bingers will experience vomiting which in turn causes many physical problems such as; torn esophagus, ripped staples lines, heart attack, stroke, malnutrition, and even death.

4. If I have to diet and exercise after having the WLS, why even have it?

Good question, one that is often asked. The WLS is a tool to lose weight, but you still have to diet and exercise. Dr. No told me I never had to worry about dieting again. Statements made by some doctors like the one I had are very misleading. Many people feel if they could lose the weight they could then exercise again and this might be true. More often than not, people will vomit to keep their weight down rather than exercise. This is especially true for those who had bulimia before the surgery.

5. Will I have to take supplements for life after the WLS?

Yes, it is essential to take supplements daily for the rest of your life. Missing them can, and does, cause long term problems, such as neuropathy from the lack of B-12. Both a naturopath and nutritionist told me the recommended amount of supplements by Dr. No was not nearly enough because of the mal-absorption. I was also told the medications I needed would have to be increased by four times because of the same problem, mal-absorption. Blood tests proved this to be true for me. I was also told by my naturopath to look for vitamins that have a high absorption rate and that are 'cold pressed' and not 'heat pressed', if taken in tablet form.

The 'heat pressed' tablets lose some of the quality of the vitamin. Check labels; ask a pharmacist, naturopath, or someone at your local heath food store for assistants. Also, look into getting B-12 shots instead of a tablet which can be given once or twice a month, depending on what your doctor recommends. Since I could not get down pills of any kind I chose the liquid form of supplements which were high in absorption, but they still weren't enough.

Everything went through me so fast, the supplements were doing very little to help me. Once I had the reversal I was able to absorb all the supplements and without taking massive amounts.

6. Will I be able to be more active after having the gastric bypass surgery?

Some people state they are able to be more active after having the surgery, but others, like me, ended up less active after the surgery.

I was in malnutrition which did not enable me to even walk across the room without struggling. I also could not go swimming without vomiting in the pool, and I was too nauseous to ride an exercise bike. There are those who have constant diarrhea and can't leave the house long enough to take a short walk without having an accident.

A few patients with this surgery stated they couldn't exercise because of a lack of iron which made them very weak. When taking large doses of iron they were nauseous and unable to leave their homes, let alone exercise. If one has problems with the WLS their physical activity will be greatly hindered.

7. Can the pouch with the gastric bypass surgery break if I eat too much?

Yes, it can and when it does it can be fatal. Patients are advised by their doctor to eat very small amounts of food. If you do eat too much or drink fluids while you eat, you will most likely vomit. But the pouch can, and does, break in some patients but it is listed as happening rarely.

8. Will I lose all my hair if I have the surgery?

A few people don't lose any of their hair, while many lose some if not all of it. Losing hair is due to the lack of nutrients. The condition of your hair is an indicator as to how your body is absorbing food and supplements.

The more malnourished you are the more your hair will fall out and look dull. It can start to grow back when you get in more food. In my case, it didn't start growing back until I had the gastric bypass reversed (or takedown). Some patients' hair never grows back as thick as it was before surgery.

9. Are there people who die from the WLS?

Yes, ASBS statistics show 1 in 1,000 people die from the surgery. However, this number could be much higher since most deaths directly linkable to the WLS are recorded as from other causes. This isn't a conspiracy but simply has something to do with the way the coroner's office words. In Sabiston: Essentials of Surgery (NY, 1994), Dr Walter Pories, a noted WLS surgeon, stated that

"The gastric bypass procedure can be performed with an operative mortality of 1 percent now" (1 death in every 100 surgeries) this text is used in medical schools.

Oftentimes, people who die from the WLS have a different reason listed as the cause of death. I was told of a patient who had severe malnutrition with organ failure, and she die. The cause of death was listed as a heart attack. It is very difficult to get accurate data on this subject and will continue to be unless the true reason is put on the death certificates. For example: A person who died from liver or kidney failure as a result of the WLS wouldn't necessarily have their death certificate list the cause of death as related to the WLS.

I noticed the people involved in the on line support groups are two years or less out from their surgery, so where are the long timers?

This is an observation many have made, including me. It could be that these people have gained back their weight and no longer fit into the cheerleading group. It could be because they now have physical problems and aren't welcome in the groups if they bring these issues up. It could also be that many of these people have died. Whatever the case may be, they are not showing up at support groups or followed by their surgeons to see how they are doing.

10. Can I still get diabetes after having the WLS?

One of the reasons people have the WLS is because they have diabetes and want to be free of it. Many who have the RNY gastric bypass surgery can have hypoglycemia because of their reaction to sugar. I never had hypoglycemia before the surgery, but did afterwards. Hypoglycemia can lead into diabetes and I was heading in that direction. While some patients will be free of diabetes after the surgery, others might develop it afterwards.

11. Are patients thoroughly informed of the pros and cons before having WLS?

It doesn't appear they are, based on the number of people who have written about the lack of information provided by their doctor and support groups before having the surgery. There is plenty of information about the pro side of WLS and very little about the con side. Every one of the people I have interviewed said they wished and deserved the down side of the surgery, and if they had this information they would not have had it.

Doctor's offices are providing lists of people who want to encourage people to have the surgery as a promotional tool, but they aren't providing lists of people with problems.

I read everything Dr. No gave me and asked several people on the list he provided, but I was a long way from being thoroughly informed.

12. Why are people who participate on the on-line support groups so hostile towards those that ask questions about the problems associated with WLS?

As far as I can tell from all the responses that I have received, these people don't want to face the fact that WLS do have problems associated with them. I should note that not all of the people on there are vicious, but the majority of them are this way, and they keep the others from speaking up. If you do speak up you will either be called bad names, ridiculed, threatened, and kicked out.

There are those that don't want to hear about problems others are having, maybe it might happen to them someday soon or already have. Nobody wants to be a failure and some do feel if they admit they have problems they have failed so keep quiet about it. A group, or sheep, mentality also exists; I want to be like everyone else so will go along with the crowd and say all is well.

The people in these groups also blame the person for having problems by not following the doctor's orders. This is so far from the truth. Why blame the victim? Offering empathy and support for those who are suffering goes a long way, but this is not happening in the majority of these groups.

People in the groups are also dispensing medical advice which should not be happening. Medical concerns should always be addressed with a qualified physician, not a lay person.

13. Will I live a longer life with the WLS?

There is no proof you will live longer with any type of WLS. It is certainly a plus to get off some weight to be healthier, but I stress the importance of getting help in finding an alternative way to be healthy without having your insides altered. You might live longer with the WLS or you might die sooner.

Some would rather die thin at all costs. The WLS is a quick fix for a long term problem. It takes less time to do surgery than it is to spend time with patients to find a way that works for them. Some doctors don't have time for individual care so surgery is often recommended.

14. Will the WLS get rid of my depression?

No, it oftentimes will get much worse after having the WLS. Dr. No told me most of his patients are on some kind of anti-depressant for life. If you suffer from depression before the surgery you will certainly have it afterwards.

Changing your outward appearance will not take care of the inner problems that need to be address fully before having any WLS. Some people feel if they are thinner they won't have any more problems and attribute their lack of self esteem due to being overweight. I would advice anyone with depression to seek out help with a therapist. Find out what the cause of the depression is before doing anything that alters the body and causes life long problems that can cause even more depression.

I never had a problem with depression before the surgery, but had severe depression after it due to malnutrition. I also suffered with anxiety disorder due to the fact I knew I was in malnutrition and felt I had no control over my health. Since the reversal all my anxiety and depression subsided.

15. Are all WLS reversible?

No, it all depends on the surgery you have and this should be discussed with your doctor before choosing the type of surgery you are considering.

The reversal is really a takedown because you can't go back exactly the way you were before the WLS.

The only surgery I know of at this time that is easier to reverse than the others forms of WLS is the Lap Band. The Lap Band still has its problems, but it is less invasive as the other methods of WLS. There have been reported deaths with the Lap Band and complications with the band around the stomach. The RNY is reversible, but it is a long and difficult procedure. Many doctors won't even consider reversing any of the weight loss surgeries.

Given the chronic problems from my RNY/Fobi it took me months to find a doctor to do the reversal. Like I said before; check out a doctor thoroughly before having them do a reversal on you. You don't want to be their first patient.

I am not advocating all people with the WLS should get it reversed, rather to think long and hard before having the surgery in the first place. You need to consider what you might have to go through later. I was informed the hospital in England reverses all the RNY procedures they performed on patients due to long term problems associated with the surgery. I personally feel all doctors should be versed in the reversal/takedown if they are doing WLS. Leaving a patient out in the cold with no where to turn for help in case they need a takedown is not right in my opinion. Many people I have received letters from can't find a doctor to do the takedown, even when they are in desperate need. It can take several months to find a qualified physician to do the takedown and who is willing to do one. Some die before they ever get the help they deserve.

30

Be Prepared

We all need to be prepared for what could go wrong and does so very often. The following is a list of the things that will help you be prepared for the surgery in the event of complications:

1. Buy lots of nightgowns because that is what you will be living in if you become too weak or sick to get dressed.

2. Be prepared to spend A LOT of money to pay out for medical care your insurance company won't pay for.

3. Hire someone to do your grocery shopping for your family.

4. If you have young children get a good nanny or child care provider to raise them.

5. Line up someone to clean your house, run errands, cook and clean, help you bath, drive you to your doctors appointments, to make

sure you are getting in enough water so you don't get dehydrated and end up in the hospital, hold your head while you cry in pain, and help you up off the floor when you fall down from malnutrition.

6. Be prepared for people who ask you if you have cancer because you look so bad.

7. Be prepared for all the tests that you will have to go through to find out why you can't keep down any food, or are weak from iron, B-12, and all the other deficiencies.

8. Be prepared for the doctor and others that will tell you all your physical problems are in your head and not in your body.

9. Get a good therapist to help you deal with the problems you will have from malnutrition. Malnutrition will cause your mind to deteriorate as well as your body.

10. Save up money to pay for all the supplements and proteins that you will have to throw away because they make you sick (lactose intolerance) or your body rejects.

11. You will have to ask your family and friends for help and take them up on it. Don't try to do more than you can or you will end up even more tired and dejected.

12. Be very prepared for your surgeon to deny you medical care and tell you to go elsewhere for help.

13. Line up a great hairdresser or wig maker to help cover the bald spots when you lose your hair.

14. Be so very prepared for those who will blame you for not following a strict diet and not taking the right kind of supplements when you know you have. It will take a bit of a tough skin to ask questions and endure attacks, called a liar even when you have done everything you were advised to do.

15. Even if you take LOTS of calcium citrate, be prepared for bone loss and osteoporosis, losing height and having bones break.

16. Be prepared if you get lupus, adhesions, cancer, bowel obstructions, intestinal blockages, and all the other maladies that are attributed to the weight loss surgery.

17. Be prepared to have your pouch burst, spewing acidic toxins throughout your body, resulting in coma and death.

18. The chronic vomiting can rip your esophagus, requiring another surgery. Also, dealing with hernias that will require surgery to repair.

19. Be prepared to stay close to a bathroom in case you have chronic vomiting or diarrhea.

20. Don't be surprised when your blood pressure goes up from the stress of problems, your cholesterol to also go up which does happen in some people, lactose intolerance, hypoglycemia, thyroid problems and more.

21. Make sure you have very good insurance that will cover long term medical care.

22. Be prepared to take more medications, higher doses might be necessary because of the mal-absorption.

23. Make sure you have a comfortable chair, couch, or bed in case you have to stay in it for long periods of time due to chronic nausea and weakness.

24. One very important issue to be prepared for is, finding a qualified doctor to do a takedown of the surgery if you have life threatening complications.

Everyone must be 'prepared' for things that can and does go wrong. This is just a few of the thing to prepare for and there are more.

31

Post Op Comments

The following are comments made from post op patients who have had a variety of weight loss surgeries (WLS); including the BPD/DS (duodenal switch), Jib (intestinal bypass), VBG (stomach stapling only, no intestinal bypass) and RNY (gastric bypass).

Support groups will list many positive comments, but I want to show the other side since these comments are left out of most lists provided by doctor's offices and group sites. It is important to look at all sides of weight loss surgery and what is happening to many patients.

Most were told problems would never happen or the risks of them having problems were so low they shouldn't even be concerned. These comments came from e-mails sent to me, personal interviews, and an on-line support group. I have been given permission to print their comments.

There is a woman who has already had a VBG, an RNY, and now going for the duodenal switch and is having problems getting insurance approval. If the first one didn't work, the second one didn't either, why have the third? I was told any of the weight loss surgeries were suppose to be permanent ways to lose weight and keep it off. Why the need for all the revisions?

My sister had the gastric bypass and thought all her problems would go away when she become thin. Wrong! She is more depressed than ever and sick all the time.

I take so much iron and it isn't doing any good. I'm still anemic.

My doctor told me I would have loose stools, but he never told me I would have to sit on the toilet all day with diarrhea. I can't go anywhere unless I wear a diaper.

The constant gas is not just a little inconvenient;; it is so bad I can clear a room in a heart beat.

I suffer from bradycardia (very slow and irregular heartbeat), the doctor feels this is from a lack of absorption of vitamins even though my levels are OK.

No one told me I would be constantly vomiting all day long, eventually ripping my esophagus and needing another surgery.

I was told my weight loss would be permanent, but I gained it all back, and for what, to be even more depressed than I was before. Not worth it!!!!!

I am hungry all the time, what is this about not having an appetite.

The honeymoon period is over for me, gained back all the weight, and then some.

Everything I eat makes me sick, I am so tired of being nauseous, and I just don't want to live anymore.

I felt altered after having the weight loss surgery; I didn't feel normal.

My surgeon told me there was little risk with the RNY and that I didn't need to worry. Ever since the surgery I have had constant diarrhea and vomiting. I suffer with malnutrition, dehydration, and vitamin deficiencies; I look like a walking skeleton. I have been in the hospital twice and the doctor said it is all in my head. I just want my life back; I'm not crazy, I'm sick.

I was told I would never have to exercise and diet again, what a crock, I eat less than I did before and still don't lose with the surgery.

I watched my friend die from her weight loss surgery and I will NEVER have one. I would rather be overweight and exercise than to be skinny and dead. I am still mourning the loss of my dear friend.

My niece is in the hospital again after having the gastric bypass three months ago. She has numbness in her stomach and legs and fell when trying to walk. She has trouble eating anything. She is now malnourished and on IVs. I am afraid she won't make it.

If I hear one more time all my problems are in my head I will throw up on my doctor. It isn't in my head, it is in my body.

Patients convey they have Lupus and cancer which were attributed to WLS.

Everyone told my friend Mona, the gastric bypass was wonderful. But now, she is in the hospital for the third time since having the surgery. She is so nauseous and can't keep in food. Everyone thinks its IN HER MIND, but I know her and that is the farthest from the truth. Now, she is very depressed.

I wanted to be thinner so I could play with my daughter and not have her end up with a fat mommy, but after having the surgery I can't even hold her. I am too weak and sick, and the doctor says he can't do anything for me. What am I to do?

I just wanted the truth about the surgery, why did my doctor lie to me, why didn't he show or tell me what does go wrong, so very wrong?

I went to the support group and left crying. They only wanted to hear the success stories and not about my regrets from having the surgery and all the ailments I now have. Where is all this help I was told would be there?

My friends say I look so old now and sick and you know what, they're right.

I have to diet and exercise even more than I did before the surgery, and I am still starving just to stay the same weight.

After two years out from my surgery I gained all the weight back and won't ever have it done again. NO revisions for me.

I am now out five years from the weight loss surgery and have gained all the weight back and a few more pounds. Now I am going to Weight Watchers and working out three times a week. Not losing, but not gaining.

I was told the surgery was a tool to lose weight, but this tool failed miserably, I only lost 30 pounds and now it is coming back on faster than ever. All the money I paid out and pain for a few pounds that won't stay off; even when I eat 1,200 calories a day.

I had done several months of research into this surgery and asked all the questions but boy was I not given everything I needed to know before making a decision. I wouldn't do it again for anything!

I have to go and have another hernia operation… When will it be over.

My doctor never told me I would never be able to have a normal meal with my family or go to a BBQ. I can't eat without running to the nearest bathroom.

My hair fell out, all of it. Where can I buy a wig?

After my friends said I looked like a walking skeleton I went home and cried. I am so tired of looking like death warmed over, just barely warmed at that.

If I hear one more celebrity tell everyone how great the gastric bypass is I will throw up, which won't be hard to do since I do that all the time. I would like them to live with me for awhile and see what it is like. They can hold my head while I vomit and clean up the diarrhea.

32

Final Comments

There is a stigma attached to people who are overweight. They are seen as less desirable, less educated, having less willpower, and discriminated against. Overweight people are often not seen as valuable assets in our society and are judged by their body size and not the size of their heart. No matter what size you are there are still many things people of all sizes can, and do, contribute to society.

People who have had the weight loss surgery are looked at by many as taking the easy way out to lose weight. They are viewed as cheaters because they didn't lose by dieting, exercising, and having willpower. Having the weight loss surgery was the hardest thing I had ever done. It's not easy to starve yourself, to vomit every day, to have chronic nausea, and to watch your life disintegrate with every day that passes.

I have often been asked if I would do it all over again to lose weight and my answer has always been the same, NO. I risked my life twice; once to have the gastric bypass and the next to have a takedown. I might have to risk it again in the future if I need further surgery from the adhesions from both surgeries. I will never again put my life at risk with any of the new and improved weight loss methods.

I will continue to work at being healthy and strong with a long term approach. Along with daily hiking I have included lifting weights.

I believe everything is possible if you want it bad enough, and feel worthy of having all you deserve. I deserve the best of health and deserve a life without life threatening problems.

I have learned through interviews with WLS patients and researching these surgeries that there are many with life threatening problems due to the surgery. For a long time I thought I was one of those rare people who was sick from the weight loss surgery, but soon found out I was not alone. There appears to be more people with problems than without. Some will dispute this statement, but if they read the stories and talk with the people that I have, they will find out how prevalent this problem really is!

Being morbidly obese does result in some serious health problems, but WLS is not the answer for most people. Overweight people do need to take control over their weight issues before taking drastic steps by altering their bodies. The weight loss surgeries will change the outside in the short-term, but does not deal with why a person gains weight.

A change in metabolism is only one reason why you can be overweight. A person needs to get a complete medical check up to make sure the weight gain isn't from a medical problem. If you're predisposed to weight gain through genetics than that is something that needs to be accepted as part of life.

No diet in the world will work, and the WLS won't work either, until a life style change is implemented. Losing weight and keeping it off are two different sets of issues. It is easier to lose weight than it is to keep it off, unless you look at why the weight came on in the first place.

Food can be a great protector, especially for those who have been abused. Those sexually abused have a higher incidence of obesity than any other group of people. If you hide behind the weight, you don't have to deal with the outside world and the comments by insensitive people. Once your internal dialogue changes, you can give yourself permission to change your outer self. Loving yourself is easier said than done for many people with weight issues, but it is essential for the healing process.

Food can be used as a medication and has been used successfully, feeding a need. Find out why and when you started medicating yourself and deal with the issue instead of burying it deeper within. Facing a painful past is a chance worth taking if you want to find out why the need for self medicating with food. Take away the need to put on weight or you will never lose it or keep it off. No amount of surgery will take care of a weight problem until the old pattern of eating is changed.

Many, people who have had WLS never dealt with the issues of why they are overweight before having the surgery so afterwards the issues are still there. They see their bodies getting smaller yet still don't feel deserving. The weight lost also comes back since the body cannot live on a small amount of food. Not all overweight people eat large amounts of food.

Many of us who have weight problems eat very little food, but are immediately judged as overeaters. Some gain weight rapidly on hormone replacements, under active thyroid, genetics, or a slow metabolism due to menopause.

When I saw my family physician at nine months out from my gastric bypass surgery I asked her, "why am I hungry all the time, is it a psychological issue or what?" She said, "It isn't psychological, it is physiological, you're not getting in enough food to live. With all the vomiting, you are not keeping in enough food. You are in a cycle of hunger and vomiting". I would be hungry and try to eat, only to vomit or become nauseous, the cycle continued day in and day out for eighteen months.

I had a long eighteen months before having the gastric bypass surgery reversed. I do deserve to be healthy and I do deserve the best quality of life I can give to myself.

Dr. No guaranteed my blood pressure would be lower, heart healthier, and cholesterol would be lower among all the other promises he made. After the surgery my blood pressure went up, my cholesterol stayed the same, and my heart was under a great deal of stress. The problems after I had the surgery were by far worse than before. Since the reversal (or takedown), all these problems have gone away and I am getting stronger by the day.

I have also started weight lifting and increased my cardiovascular work outs. Now I can do what I did before having the gastric bypass surgery. During those eighteen months with the surgery my muscles had atrophied, and now I will work at getting my body back into shape.

I also am able to get in enough food so I can work out. This not only helps my body, it does wonders for my spirit. I don't exercise to lose weight but to make me feel better. If I hadn't decided to fight for my life, I would still be lying in bed suffering. I was not going to take no for an answer when looking for help. I had a great deal of support to get me through those difficult times and will be forever grateful to so many.

My family and friends see my happiness return and are so excited for me. The surgical specialist I saw for my reversal three months' check-up told me I don't need to come back unless I have a problem. For now, I have a clean bill of health to do whatever I want.

Part of what I want to accomplish with this book is to help people make an informed decision. Know what can and does go wrong will help determine if the risk is worth it. It will take a lot of thought if a person wants to trade one set of problems for another. I also wrote this book to work through what I went through in order to heal myself and move on. I will continue to address peoples concerns and answer questions. I have started to rebuild my company and have enough energy to do much more.

Some days are hard to get through when I receive several letters from people who have problems related to their weight loss surgery. My heart goes out to them. I have heard from friends and family members who are concerned about their loved ones. I can relate to these people because I've been there and know how important it is to have someone to talk with.

I will direct people to others who can help them, to a doctor who is well-versed in the treatment of problems associated with weight loss surgeries, and to those who are willing to listen. Sometimes being there for someone who is in pain, medically or emotionally, is all a person needs at that point in time.

A good support group can be very valuable in the healing process. A group that is without judgment allows each person to bring up all issues pertaining to their weight loss surgery. I want everyone to be in the best health possible, no matter what choice they made regarding weight loss surgery.

Since the reversal, I do not have any guilt about what I eat. Food is my friend and I will put into my body food that gives me the ability to become strong. I have taken back control of my life and won't ever give that away to anyone again. I chose to have the gastric bypass surgery to save my life and when that didn't work I made the choice to reverse it. The healing process for me began once I said, "I Want To Live". The first step had been taken, and now the rest fell into place. There will be no more punishing of my body. I embrace who I am and the body I have.

I do feel many people are unhappy with their weight and want to be thinner than they are, even if they are not severely obese. Many people try to make their bodies achieve an ideal weight or desired shape by punishing themselves. They may lose weight and feel successful for a while, but eventually most of these people fail and end up even more unhappy with themselves. These people have tried to start by changing their bodies first. Your body cannot be separated from you self-image. When you start at the beginning, you need to develop a complete and positive concept of yourself. You need to be at peace with yourself, to like yourself and others, and to treat yourself with love, not punishment. Your physical being does not take its shape directly from what you do to it, that is, from what you eat or how you exercise. Many people have gone through starvation and still didn't lose weight. The physical self responds to the attitude you have of your body. Once your self-image improves, you can begin to reduce the inner pressure put on yourself and free your body of its outer fat. Your body is at the effect of your mind and your mind rules your body. When you change your thinking and attitude, your weight and appearance will change. Once you learn to love yourself for the way you are you can become the self you want to be.

My life has come full circle and I get the chance to help anyone who asks for it. "I Want To Live" was the words I spoke when I wanted more out of my life. I will continue to help others who "want to live" and fight for their lives.

33

References

Sue Widemark's Information Site on WLS:
http://gastricbypass.netfirms.com

Sue Widemark's Weight Loss Surgery Support Group:
WLS_uncensored@yahoogroups.com

"Surgery For Weight Loss Comparisons Of Risk and
Benefit" by Paul Ernsberger, PhD. From Obesity
Health (renamed Healthy Weight Journal) March-April
1991, pp. 24-25

Wooley, Susan C: "The Psychological and Social
Aspects of Obesity"-Bender, A et al: Body Weight
Control, (London, 1991)

The Alvarado Clinic: http://gastricbypass.com

National Institute of Mental Health (NIMH)
Office of Communications and Public Liaison

Public Inquiries: (301) 443-4513
Media Inquiries: (301) 443-4536
E-mail: nimhinfo@nih.gov
Web site: http://eatingdisorders.about.com

American Society for Bariatric Surgery (ASBS)
http://www.asbs.org/

Pacific Institute of Surgery for Obesity
http://www.pacificsurgery.com

About The Author

Dani is a college educated woman with her own business. She has been interviewed for several articles and appeared on national television to discuss the pros and cons of gastric bypass surgery.

Dani has been married to her husband for 28 years and has twin sons. She is also an identical twin. Dani's sisters, brothers and mother support her decision to come forward in telling her experience with the weight loss surgery and its' reversal.

Although Dani is a very private person she felt it was important to tell what she went through with the surgery in order to inform others about the risks of the weight loss surgery and what does go wrong. She knew there were others like herself that suffered in silence with their complications and wanted to reach out to them.

Dani answers letters and phone calls on a daily basis from people seeking help, understanding, and compassion relating to weight loss surgery (WLS).

For over 24 years Dani has been a practitioner of the healing arts. She shares her knowledge of her Native American spirituality with those who wish to learn more about the 'red path' and the ways of the Goddess Mother Earth.

Dani loves to learn and is a determined person to make positive changes in her life. She encourages others to follow their hearts and to realize the gifts they have within are special.